HIT
or Miss

Lessons Learned from Health Information Technology Implementations

Editor
Jonathan Leviss, MD

Associate Editors
Pam Charney, PhD, RD
Christopher Corbit, MD
Justin Graham, MD, MS
Brian Gugerty, DNS, MS, RN
Bonnie Kaplan, PhD
Gail Keenan, PhD, RN
Larry Ozeran, MD
Eric Poon, MD, MPH
Eric Rose, MD
Scot Silverstein, MD
Edward Wu, MD

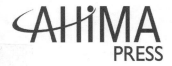

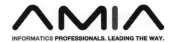

ISBN 978-1-58426-397-5

AHIMA Product No. AB102213

AHIMA Staff:
Jessica Block, MA, Assistant Editor
Jason O. Malley, Director, Creative Content Development
Ashley Sullivan, Production Development Editor

For more information about AHIMA Press publications, including updates, visit http://www.ahima.org/publications/updates.aspx.

American Health Information Management Association
233 North Michigan Avenue, 21st Floor
Chicago, Illinois 60601-5800
ahima.org

AMIA aims to lead the way in transforming healthcare through trusted science, education, and the practice of informatics. AMIA connects a broad community of professionals and students interested in informatics. AMIA is the bridge for knowledge and collaboration across a continuum, from basic and applied research to the consumer and public health arenas.

AMIA
4720 Montgomery Lane, Suite 500
Bethesda, Maryland 20814
amia.org

To Rebecca and Emily—Explore, fail,
learn…and enjoy it all!

To Perri—My wife, most treasured colleague, and best
friend. Thanks for your encouragement, criticism,
sense of adventure, and love. Much aloha.

To my friends, family, and colleagues—Thanks for sharing
successes and failures and for not focusing too much on either.

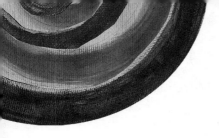

Contents

PART I: Hospital Care Focus

PART III: Community Focus

PART IV: Conclusion

PART V: Appendices

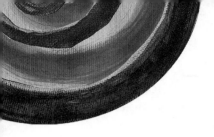

About the Editors and Contributors

Volume Editor

Jonathan A. Leviss, MD

Jonathan Leviss is the Chief Medical Officer of the Rhode Island Quality Institute (RIQI); he provides physician leadership across initiatives to improve the quality, safety, and value of healthcare in Rhode Island, including the statewide Beacon Community Program and Health Information Exchange (HIE). He is a Clinical Assistant Professor of Health Services, Policy & Practice at the Warren Alpert Medical School of Brown University. Previously, Dr. Leviss was Vice President, Chief Medical Officer at Sentillion through its acquisition by Microsoft, where he served as Director, Clinical Solutions, in the Microsoft Health Solutions Group. Dr. Leviss was the first CMIO at the New York City Health and Hospitals Corporation and was medical school faculty at NYU and Columbia University. He practices as an internist at the Thundermist Health Center in Rhode Island.

Associate Editors

Christopher Corbit, MD

Christopher Corbit is the Chief Medical Informatics Officer at Emergency Medicine Physicians. He was a Fellow for the National Library of Medicine, Medical Informatics Course in 2005. He is board certified in Emergency Medicine and is a fellow of the American College of Emergency Physicians.

Justin V. Graham, MD, MS

Justin Graham is Chief Medical Information Officer for NorthBay Health System in Fairfield, California. He is a nationally recognized leader in the practical realities of transforming clinical practice using healthcare IT and the electronic health record. Dr. Graham is board certified in infectious diseases and holds a master's degree in biomedical informatics. He trained at UCSF, Harvard, and Stanford.

Brian Gugerty, DNS, MS, RN

Brian Gugerty is CEO of GIC Informatics, a clinical informatics consulting firm specializing in physician-to-physician electronic health record activation support and evaluation of healthcare information technology. Brian is active in AMIA and has authored or coauthored over forty articles and book chapters on informatics topics.

Bonnie Kaplan, PhD, FACMI

Bonnie Kaplan chairs the AMIA People and Organizational Issues and the Ethical, Legal, and Social Issues Working Groups and is a fellow of the American College of Medical Informatics. She is faculty at Yale University and the University of Illinois at Chicago. Her consulting and research involves people's reactions to new technologies in healthcare and evaluating applications of information systems, for which she received the AMIA President's Award in 2000.

Gail Keenan, PhD, RN

Gail Keenan is an Associate Professor and the Director of the Nursing Informatics Initiative at the University of Illinois-Chicago College of Nursing. Gail has been actively involved in health informatics education, research, and policy for more than a decade. Her research has focused on ensuring the usability and interoperable representation of nursing in the electronic health record. She has received NIH and AHRQ R01 funding awards to support her research and has published multiple related manuscripts.

Larry Ozeran, MD

Larry Ozeran is President of Clinical Informatics and advises clients on public policy, strategic planning, provider engagement, and clinician training. He works with many organizations, including CalOHI, Cal eConnect, and CalHIPSO, serving in leadership capacities with the national associations AMDIS, AMIA, and HIMSS. He received an award from the State of California for his HIT contributions. Larry is a practicing general surgeon.

Eric G. Poon, MD, MPH

Eric Poon is Vice President and Chief Medical Information Officer at Boston Medical Center, MA, where he leads the implementation of the new EHR and analytics strategy. Eric previously served as the Director of Clinical Informatics at Brigham and Women's Hospital, overseeing the development and implementation of clinical systems.

Eric Rose, MD, FAAFP

Eric Rose is a practicing family physician with eight years' experience in development of commercial clinical information system applications and content. He is a graduate of the Albert Einstein College of Medicine and a Fellow of the American Academy of Family Physicians. He is on the faculty of the Departments of Family Medicine and Biomedical and Health Informatics at the University of Washington School of Medicine.

Scot Silverstein, MD

Scot Silverstein completed a medical informatics fellowship at Yale and was then faculty. He was CMIO at a large hospital in Delaware and was director of the science libraries and The Merck Index at Merck. Currently at Drexel University, he teaches, writes, and provides expert witness services regarding health IT.

Edward Wu, MD

Edward Wu is Director of Physician Services at Dearborn Advisors. His expertise is in clinician adoption of information technology across multiple practice environments. He has led multiple CPOE implementations and quality initiatives for healthcare organizations. He continues to experience the "joy of CPOE" as a practicing hospitalist.

Contributing Case Authors

The editors and publishers would like to thank the following people for contributing the original case studies included in this book. Following is an alphabetical listing of the authors (and author teams).

- Jeffrey M. Adams, PhD, RN; Audrey Parks, MBA; and Virginia I. Williams, MSN, RN (coauthors)
- Lawrence B. Afrin, MD; Frank Clark, PhD; John Waller, MD; Patrick Cawley, MD; Timothy Hartzog, MD; Mark Daniels, MS; and Deborah Campbell, RN (coauthors)
- Pam Charney, PhD, RD
- Christopher Corbit, MD
- Chris Doyle, MD
- Wen Dombrowski, MD
- Justin Graham, MD, MS
- Brian Gugerty, DNS, MS, RN
- Christopher Harle, PhD; Marvin Dewar, MD, JD; and Laura Gruber, MBA, MHS (coauthors)
- Melinda Jenkins, PhD, FNP
- Bonnie Kaplan, PhD
- Gail Keenan, PhD, RN

- Christoph Lehmann, MD; Roberto A. Romero, BS; and George R. Kim, MD (coauthors)
- Jonathan Leviss, MD
- Steven Magid, MD
- Sandi Mitchell, BS Pharm, MSIS
- Ilene Moore, MD
- Kenneth Ong, MD, MPH
- Larry Ozeran, MD
- Patrick A. Palmieri, EdS, MBA, MSN, ACNP, RN
- Liron Pantanowitz, MD and Anil V. Parwani, MD, PhD (coauthors)
- Eric Poon, MD, MPH
- Brad Rognrud, MS, RPh
- Eric Rose, MD
- Robert Schwartz, MD
- Scot Silverstein, MD
- Diane Stevens, RN
- Walton Sumner, MD and Phil Asaro, MD
- Vivian Vimarlund, Bahlol Rahimi, and Toomas Timpka (coauthors)
- Riikka Vuokko, Anne Forsell, and Helena Karsten (coauthors)
- Edward Wu, MD

CMIO Musings were contributed by Steven Magid, MD and Jonathan Leviss, MD.

Graphics

Amy Lash Boyes

Amy Lash Boyes grew up south of Boston, spending much of her time painting, sailing, and enjoying the outdoors. With a fine arts degree, she worked as a graphic designer for nine years at a firm and now is a freelance graphics designer and artist. Amy created the graphics seen throughout HIT or Miss, 2nd Edition.

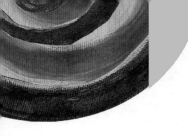

Acknowledgments

This book exists because of the team effort of the editors, the support of the AMIA Clinical Information Systems Working Group, the information sharing with our colleagues about many failed—and successful—HIT initiatives, and the professional guidance, editing, and commitment of the AHIMA publishing team.

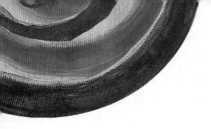

Foreword

When the first volume of HIT *or Miss* came out three years ago, many of us carried it around like college students of the 1950s with their copies of *Lady Chatterley's Lover*. HIT *or Miss* contained what few uttered out loud but what all knew to be essential, basic, and true. Implementing health information technology (HIT) was difficult, often precarious, and always involved uncertain outcomes. Nevertheless, most of us felt and still feel the promise of HIT is so great that it was (and is) worth the effort. The first edition of HIT *or Miss* did not say the emperor was entirely naked, but it exposed the threadbare reality faced by medical offices and hospitals implementing and using HIT. It told us what we increasingly understood: HIT is a magnificent idea but its execution was generally a serious struggle—most often a struggle each hospital or office negotiated alone. There was little cross learning, little knowledge transfer. As the saying goes: "You've seen one EHR implementation, you've seen one EHR implementation." Sometimes the systems worked, often they did not; always, it took a lot more work than could be imagined.

In a recent advertisement for one of the Healthcare Information and Management Systems Society (HIMSS) webinars (Novak 2012), HIMSS noted that "IT Projects Have a 70% Failure Rate…" and offered project-management training as a solution. Ordinarily, an admission of that high a failure rate would generate condemnation from HIMSS and the Office of the National Coordinator for Health Information Technology (ONC), accusing those voicing such heresy of technophobia, Luddite tendencies, and worse. What the industry promoters still fail to understand is that we learn far more from examining our mistakes than from touting our successes—especially when those successes may obscure myriad problems that were (successfully) surmounted. One of the joys of this second edition of HIT *or Miss* is that it continues to move us up on the learning curve from the official presentation of HIT as the "Happy Buddha" to the reality of what must be done to get HIT to work *in situ*. It shows us that denying the desire for interoperability, or for usable displays of lab reports, or for responsive vendors, or for sensible drop-down menus will not achieve nirvana—but will just give us more patient-safety dangers and continuing clinical inefficiencies. Nor will contentment arrive with the next upgrade. We are more likely to reach some satisfaction when we recognize the need for constant vigilance and evaluation by our clinical and information technology (IT) personnel, along with cooperation from vendors and regulators. That is where this book is so valuable. Achieving usable HIT requires we learn from these remarkably clear and thoughtful examples. I am unequivocal that each chapter offers invaluable lessons on HIT's implementation and use. Some focus on computerized physician order entry (CPOE); some on bar coding; some on electronic health records (EHRs); some on medication reconciliation; most on workflow; almost all on the need for planning and how planning is never enough; many on the understanding of HIT as transformative rather than just a tool; most on the need for constant review and evaluation. In fact, several of the chapters speak of the vision and synoptic understanding required for HIT to work. We learn also that we are never done: upgrades and patches are a river of tasks; connections with the many other systems are vulnerabilities as well as opportunities; our clinicians need training on changes; if we are a teaching hospital, we face additional challenges of HIT training while teaching patient care; all facilities face new users of varying skill levels; almost all facilities confront users with experiences of other systems (ongoing or past) with very different interfaces and ways of finding essential data; and such; and such.

The Role of the ONC, Meaningful Use, and Getting Systems to Work

Many of these chapters discuss efforts to achieve regulatory compliance. The background for this—and a source of significant criticism—is ONC's emphasis on purchasing HIT rather than on improving HIT such that we'd want to buy it. Many, also, are incensed at ONC's refusal to oblige vendors to develop or adopt data format standards and interoperability as the bases of meaningful HIT software. To be fair, ONC's and CMS's new, second iterations of "meaningful use" (MU2) regulations for 2014 are a serious move in the right direction. While many of us wanted these standards and regulations years ago, I heartily praise this very positive direction. Moreover, it is true that setting national standards requires consideration of the ocean of incompatible systems that have developed over the past many years. For example, a lot of systems must interact with laboratories or pharmacies that are only recently incorporating full digital communications. Equally true—and unfortunate—my informal survey of hospital IT systems found that hospitals had as many as 150 major IT systems and a few hundred more minor IT systems. Alas, many of these systems do not communicate with each other or with the core HIT systems (EHRs, CPOE, pharmacy IT, electronic medication administration records (eMARs), and such). There, again, we face the Tower of Babel we relish as modern medical technology. We can ask why the vendors were allowed to create such chaos. But the issue here is our efforts to make these systems work together for the benefit of patients. Implementation, thus, as so well described by these authors, is more than getting *one* system to work; it is getting many IT systems to work together…while each is undergoing change from vendors, users, and the interplay with others' systems.

The lack of standards, and the significant challenges their absence engenders, are not new to healthcare and certainly not new to industry. The United States has faced such problems before: we had dozens of railroad gauges, hundreds of time zones, and even areas with both left- and right-hand driving rules. In all cases, the federal government established standards, and the people, the economy, and especially the resistant industries flourished. Claims by industry that such standards would restrict innovation were turned on their heads. There is a lesson here for HIT vendors and for regulators. Many of the tales told in these chapters would be shorter and more pleasant if the lack of data standards and interoperability had been confronted earlier.

I once testified before the HIT Policy Committee that each medical office and each hospital implements HIT the way teenagers learn about relationships: with much uncertainty, a lot of dubious advice, and many unfortunate consequences. The teens, however, are blessed with remarkable user interfaces and usability evolved over millions of years. Before HIT *or* Miss existed, there were, of course, efforts to tell the real tales of HIT and help neophytes. But unhappy reports were usually spurned as the ravings of malcontents. HIT *or* Miss's first edition was a needed guide for those seeking to implement HIT, which was of course best accomplished with the knowledge only learned from others' real experiences (or, from our own). The first edition provided some of that. With this second edition, we have more guidance from more examples and greater insights. The editorial comments continue to be models of brevity and clear thinking.

The argument about whether or not HIT is better than paper is silly. HIT is better than paper. It is also better than wet clay slabs with cuneiform styluses, pigeons, or smoke signals. The task we face is implementing HIT in ways that work reasonably well, and then using HIT to better serve patients and clinicians. HIT *or* Miss's second edition is just what the doctor needs, and should order stat.

Ross Koppel, PhD
University of Pennsylvania

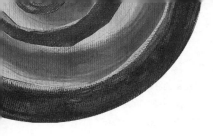

Introduction
and Methodology

Introduction

(J. Leviss and L. Ozeran)

On February 24, 2009, President Barack Obama pledged to the entire United States Congress, "Our...plan will invest in electronic health records and new technology that will reduce errors, bring down costs, ensure privacy, and save lives" (Obama 2009).

President Obama declared that digitizing healthcare will be a critical success factor in improving healthcare in the United States and the overall US economy. Through the American Recovery and Reinvestment Act of 2009 (ARRA), the federal government offered large-scale funding to create a technology foundation for the US healthcare delivery system. The ARRA's electronic health record (EHR) "Meaningful Use" program has already awarded billions of dollars to physicians and hospitals and even more will be spent in the upcoming years. The ARRA expenditure also correlates to billions of dollars spent on health information technology (HIT) software, hardware, and consulting services, all with the goal of improving the quality and efficiency of healthcare.

But what has occurred so far? Many large and small healthcare organizations have successfully leveraged the ARRA funding opportunity to advance into the digital age, but many others have faltered. Innumerable anecdotes report the high frequency with which healthcare providers and vendors fail to follow recognized best practices for HIT implementation, whether at an organization that is new to HIT or an experienced organization that is implementing a new technology. Regularly shared struggles to achieve Meaningful Use accreditation by many hospitals and physician practices raise concerns about our readiness to advance to Stage 2 and Stage 3 on a national scale in the time frame allotted by the Meaningful Use program. Why are these problems occurring? How can we learn from these problems to successfully implement HIT and advance our healthcare delivery systems into the modern digital age of other industries?

Each sequential EHR Meaningful Use stage corresponds to advancing criteria of functionality and adoption. Meaningful Use Stage 1 focuses on data capturing and sharing, but most requirements have low thresholds of adoption and do not require broad impact on the practices of most health-care professionals, even those who successfully attest (for example, the computerized physician order entry (CPOE) requirement is only for 30 percent of patients and is met with at least one medication). The successful attestation for Stage 1 does not mean that a hospital or physician practice is ready to expand the same functionality across its entire organization. Stage 2 expands upon the accomplishments of Stage 1 with requirements for advanced clinical processes but still with low adoption thresholds (such as EHR reminders for preventive care for 10 percent of patients). Stage 2 accreditation, therefore, gets more complex and involves broader aspects of a healthcare organization, but again does not require a full commitment to digitize care within a physician practice or across a major medical center. As a result, hospitals and practices can and are developing strategies to digitize parts of their organizations in order to achieve accreditation and receive the ARRA payments, without needing to support full-scale transformation to digital healthcare.

Meaningful Use Stage 3 will require measuring the clinical care and results, addressing shortcomings, and improving clinical outcomes. Also, according to the Office of the National Coordinator for Health Information Technology (ONC) draft proposal, providers and health systems must accomplish broad adoption of complex technologies (for example, CPOE rates must exceed 60 percent of all orders and medication administration must be digitized). (At the time of publication, the EHR Meaningful Use Stage 3 program had not been finalized and only draft recommendations for the requirements had been published by the ONC.) Importantly, most of the healthcare quality and cost saving benefits HIT promises require achieving Meaningful Use Stage 3. Therefore, Stage 3 accreditation, and the return on investment for the federal government's HIT investment, will first require large scale successful and sustainable rollouts of technologies that only needed to be "piloted" for Stages 1 and 2; achieving success in Stage 1 and Stage 2 does not necessarily prepare us for Stage 3.

Some cases to consider:

A hospitalized patient's INR (blood clotting time) becomes dangerously elevated; an investigation finds that the patient received double doses of anticoagulant medication due to an error in how the medication order was processed by the pharmacy computer system after being entered by the CPOE system. (Chapter 8)

A multisite fifty-provider ambulatory care organization is live on an EHR for two years—all demographic and clinical processes are completely dependent on the EHR and its practice management system, including patient registration, test results review, CPOE, and clinical documentation. One day, the EHR develops slow response times and in a few hours becomes unusable. (Chapter 28)

An ICU patient receives a medication and has an anaphylactic response—root cause analysis identifies that the pharmacy system–medication cabinet interface was scheduled for downtime when the incident occurred. Without the usual safety systems in place, a nurse had administered a similarly spelled but different medication from that ordered. (Chapter 9)

A medical center recruits and hires a physician at 80 percent time to be the CPOE go-live leader—chair the governance committees, spearhead communications about CPOE, and oversee the design, build, and rollout of CPOE. Without sufficient support for a full CMIO role, the physician becomes overwhelmed and leaves. Without formal leadership, the initiative has significant delays and fails to deliver the original functionality of the CPOE system. (Chapter 21)

What defines failure? For the purposes of discussion, we, the editorial team of HIT *or* Miss, define a health information technology (HIT) failure as "a case in which an unintended negative consequence occurred, such as a project delay, a substantial cost overrun, a failure to meet an intended goal or objective, or complete abandonment of the project."

HIT projects fail at a rate up to 70 percent of the time (Kaplan 2009). What happens when HIT projects fail? What will happen when the same hospitals or physician practices that struggled to meet Meaningful Use Stage 1 are unable to meet Stage 2 or Stage 3? What will happen when scarce healthcare dollars are spent on projects that do not meet the intended goals? Or when patients are harmed as a result of failed HIT projects? How do health systems and individual providers analyze the costs, challenges, and patient safety problems from such failed initiatives?

The editors of this book have led successful EHR and HIT projects that brought readily available patient and health information to all points of healthcare delivery and offered the types of benefits Meaningful Use Stages 2 and 3 were modeled upon. As a group, we are both excited and concerned by the potential outcomes of the ARRA funding. Although ARRA addresses the financial burden of HIT investments, many other challenges remain for successful HIT projects and the success of the EHR Meaningful Use program.

The content and human factors associated with implementing technology have proven to be formidable barriers impeding the widely available transformation that HIT could bring. Moreover, the same lessons or "best practices" required for successful HIT projects are being repeatedly learned through trial and error, over and over again, in large and small health systems without successful dissemination of the knowledge across organizations and at great financial cost and social cost. Professional conferences routinely share experiences from successful HIT initiatives, but the lessons do not appear to follow the new technologies to other organizations or update over time—the common errors remain common.

Sharing success stories does not work, or as William Soroyan wrote, "Good people are good because they've come to wisdom through failure. We get very little wisdom from success, you know" (Saroyan 1971). Apparently in the field of HIT, we do "not know." As a result, the adoption of effective HIT remains at a fairly primitive stage compared with IT adoption in every other major industry.

This collection of HIT case studies offers an approach to change the current HIT knowledge paradigm. The book contains expert insight into key remaining obstacles that must be overcome to leverage IT in order to modernize and transform healthcare. The purpose of reporting HIT case studies that failed is to document, catalogue, and share key lessons that all project managers of HIT, health system leaders in informatics and technology, hospital executives, policy makers, and service and technology providers must know in order to succeed with HIT, a critical step for the transformation of all health systems.

HIT *or Miss* presents a model to discuss HIT failures in a safe and protected manner, providing an opportunity to focus on the lessons offered by a failed initiative as opposed to worrying about potential retribution for exposing a project as having failed. Learning from failures is what every major industry regularly does. Air travel safety is enabled by organizations like the Commercial Aviation Safety Team (CAST), a multidisciplinary coalition of government and industry experts that analyzes accidents and safety incidents for continued safety improvements; mountaineers famously read the journal *Accidents in North American Mountaineering* to learn about the devastating errors of their peers and avoid repeating them; and business developers scrutinize failed efforts, from the failed solar energy company Solyndra to Apple's early handheld device, the Newton. Clinical departments around the world learn from failures in regularly scheduled "morbidity and mortality" rounds.

At the American Medical Informatics Association (AMIA) 2006 Fall Conference, the Clinical Information Systems Working Group (CIS-WG) hosted an "open-microphone" event called "Tales from the Trenches" where members shared HIT failures from their own institutions. The "Tales From the Trenches" event, created for professional development and entertainment purposes, quickly proved the value of sharing failure cases and lessons learned in a safe and protected environment. A group of us committed to publishing a collection of brief vignettes that documented situations that did not go quite right, but could be generalized so a larger audience would learn from the collective wisdom of these stories rather than repeat the same (often costly) mistakes. We committed to deidentifying all aspects of the submissions prior to publication and all submitting authors agreed to have their names appear in the book, separate and not linked to their case submissions. The unanimous agreement among all contributing authors to have their names listed in the both the first and second editions of HIT *or Miss* reinforces the message that reviewing failed initiatives offers valuable knowledge and insight, rather than an opportunity for casting blame and defensive posturing.

You will find these case studies catalogued by HIT project (such as CPOE, ambulatory EHR, and so on), but the index will also allow you to search based upon types of lessons learned (such as project management, technology failure, and so on). The catalogue and index should enable you, the reader, to find the right anecdote that best applies to your specific circumstance to present to others in your organization. The storytelling format is intended to make it easier for you to reach out to peers, superiors, and staff to say "this could be us" and then to proactively address problems before they spiral out of control.

Learning from failures is an iterative process. Do not permit all of the cost of failure to be borne by your organization. Instead, reflect on these failures as if they occurred in your circumstance so that you can improve your organization's chances of success and reduce your risk of financial and social loss. We trust that you will find this collection to be a useful guide in your efforts. With effective knowledge sharing, we can successfully lead healthcare into the digital age.

Methodology

All cases published in HIT *or Miss*, 2nd edition were voluntarily submitted by authors who were directly involved in the projects themselves; 17 cases were accepted and published in the first volume of HIT *or Miss* and an additional 17 cases were accepted for the second edition, which includes all 34 cases. Prior to the first edition of HIT *or Miss*, the editorial team agreed upon the definition of HIT failure:

> An HIT *project failure is one in which an unintended negative consequence occurred such as a project delay, a substantial cost overrun, failure to meet an intended goal or objective, or abandonment of the project.*

Requests for deidentified cases that met the definition were solicited from various professional society listservs and other professional networking. All submissions were carefully reviewed by the editorial team for publication. The editorial team assumed ultimate responsibility for reviewing, organizing, editing, and deidentifying the case material, and for providing additional expert commentary. All submitting authors of cases attested to participation in the described HIT project and the originality of the work. All cases were deidentified, removing all names of locations, organizations, and vendors, as well as identifying descriptions that were not essential to the lessons offered by the case. All opinions and analyses of the authors and editors are purely their own and do not necessarily reflect the opinions of the other authors or editors of HIT *or Miss*, AMIA, or AHIMA.

Part I
Hospital Care Focus

Six Blind Sages and the EHR

If six blind sages approached an EHR, like the elephant, the observations would vary greatly. An EHR could be observed to enhance communications, improve efficiency, standardize practices, or improve health care quality and safety. Each observation would be valid. However, each serves different masters (or end-users) whose needs must be understood and respected. Failure to agree on an overall goal for an EHR, to recognize the "animal" in its entirety, prevents problems from being managed or conflicts from being overcome.

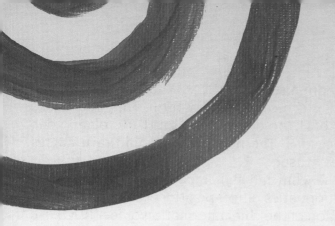

Build It with Them, Make It Mandatory, and They Will Come: Implementing CPOE

Editor: Bonnie Kaplan

Key Words:	Project Categories:	Lessons Learned Categories:
change management, computerized provider order entry (CPOE), go-live support, pilot	computerized provider order entry (CPOE), inpatient electronic health record (EHR)	implementation approaches, leadership/ governance

 Case Study

Middle Health System (Middle) has a 650-bed "downtown" hospital, a 350-bed suburban hospital, a 160-bed rehabilitation hospital, and two rural hospitals with 75 to 100 beds. They have 20 other divisions, including a 100-provider medical practice and a visiting nurse business.

Over 15 years, Middle had steady improvements in automation of many business and clinical processes, and then entered another phase, the "clinician high impact" phase of health information technology (HIT). They would acquire and implement new modules of their main vendor's electronic health record (EHR) in their inpatient settings: computerized provider order entry

(CPOE), bar code medication administration (BCMA), advanced nursing documentation, and then physician clinical documentation. This would take physicians from occasional users of HIT to dependence on HIT to plan, order, document, and make clinical decisions. The new system would take nurses from moderate users of HIT to heavy users.

CPOE was the first module in the "clinician high impact" phase to be implemented. Middle's chief medical informatics officer position was vacant, so the HIT project came under the direction of the chief information officer (CIO). He was aware of two common recommendations of those who have implemented CPOE:

- "Make CPOE use mandatory."
- "Implement CPOE throughout the enterprise."

However, the CIO thought that mandating use of CPOE was "all well and good for university medical centers," where the ratio of residents to physicians is high. Residents are younger and thus more comfortable with computers; in addition, they are under the direction of their superiors and can be ordered to perform certain tasks. His organization had 50 residents and 1,000 hospitalists, surgeons, midlevel providers, and community doctors. It was unrealistic, he thought, to mandate CPOE. His thinking was, "Build it right, and they will come."

The CPOE planning team also decided on a pilot approach. To mitigate the risk of confusion with a combination of paper and electronic orders, the two nursing units in the suburban hospital that had the fewest transfers from or into other units were chosen as the pilot units.

Despite adequate training of providers and more than adequate support during go-live, several physicians avoided using CPOE on the pilot units from the start. These physicians phoned in their orders so as not to be "harassed" by the bevy of CPOE go-live support staff. Most providers at least tolerated the system but many of those complained of the increased time it took to write orders. Several physicians on the pilot units confided to project team members that they were just "playing along" with the CPOE and were not truly supportive of the change. "If it fails, it will go away, so I don't need to learn it," said one physician who continued to write orders with a pen.

At day 16, 66 percent of the orders were created via CPOE. A successful pilot was declared. Several of the key players on the CPOE team took vacations. The project manager took two weeks off. Upon her return, she discovered that only 15 percent of the orders were being placed by CPOE. Out of concern for patient safety issues in a mixed CPOE and paper order environment, CPOE was discontinued on the pilot units two weeks later.

Following are the key lessons learned from the Middle Health System case.

- *Change management is at least as important as technical management, process transformation, and other critical aspects of a CPOE project.* Many people resist change in general. Most clinicians really resist change to their core processes to plan, order, and document care, which a CPOE implementation directly affects. A strong change management plan should be created and executed for a CPOE project.

- *Make CPOE use mandatory for all providers who write orders.* To keep providers from getting around this requirement, have all orders that are not entered directly by CPOE go through a predetermined process, such as the Joint Commission telephone order read-back procedure: a nurse logs onto the system, retrieves information for the patient in question, enters the order the provider wants, and reads it back to the provider. Because this process takes at least twice as long as the provider ordering directly into the computer via CPOE, providers quickly learn to enter their own orders.

- *Don't call it a "pilot." Consider using a rapid multiphase implementation of CPOE.* Many of the physicians involved regarded the pilot as a tryout of CPOE rather than the beginning of CPOE. You want to give the strong message that phase 1 of implementation is where users learn and then apply the lessons to other units, after a period of consolidation. Through dialogue with clinicians throughout the planning and implementation phases, clear understanding of the benefits and costs of CPOE to not only the organization but to individual organizational members should develop so that people are thinking and saying, "It's here to stay, so I'd better learn it."

- *Don't withdraw CPOE go-live support too quickly.* A user is comfortable after entering orders on approximately 30 patients. A high-volume order writer might write orders on 15 patients per week and thus will have reached the first plateau of competent use of CPOE in about two weeks. A low-volume order writer might write orders on one or two patients a week. You may have to keep some scaled-down go-live support for up to six months for low-volume order writers.

Editor's Commentary

It is not unusual for initial enthusiasm or usage to taper off. Two weeks is too short a time for a change to become institutionalized. Many problems can occur in the first few weeks without warranting discontinuing an implementation, and apparent successes can occur without warranting that all is well. Sustained support, reinforcement, and evaluating what is happening are needed to maintain a desired trajectory.

Attention should have been paid to early indicators that there could be problems. Not all providers were willing to use the system so as to avoid what they considered "harassment" by the support staff. Others "at least tolerated the system" but complained that it took longer to write orders. Some even confided that they were not supportive of the change, but were "playing along." None of these issues were addressed. If it would take longer to enter orders, physicians would need to understand why CPOE was important. Perhaps the time it takes to enter orders would decrease as staff learned better how to use the system, in which case they should have been helped both to understand the learning curve and to grasp concepts more quickly. Training, however, was described as "at least adequate" when it could have been better than minimally sufficient.

Different user communities, such as nurses and physicians, will have different incentives, training and support needs, attitudes, and aptitudes that need addressing. The benefits of using the system, or at least reasons why it should be used even if there are no obvious benefits to the users, also need to be highlighted and reinforced.

The pilot units were chosen because they had a low volume of transfers. The case study does not indicate how these units were viewed by the rest of the organization or whether there were other characteristics that could have affected what developed. A positive experience with the first units where change is implemented will serve as a good example to other units. In addition to selecting a test bed that is not too challenging, as was done here, other considerations include whether people on the unit might be respected project champions and if there is strong leadership support in the unit for the project.

Another issue is that several key players took vacation at the same time, very early in the implementation. Although the vacation time was likely well deserved, having several key players gone at the same time meant there were not enough people available to notice and address the developing problem of nonuse of CPOE. Mechanisms to assess progress and take steps to alleviate problematic developments before they got out of hand should have been in place. Especially in the early days of implementation, it can be quite helpful to continue with training efforts as unfamiliar situations are encountered, and also to monitor where things do not go smoothly, where workarounds are occurring, and where complaints are developing. It appears there was no such plan in place, and without key people on site, there was no ad hoc means of addressing emerging issues. As a result, an early success quickly turned into an early failure.

 Lessons Learned

- Change management is critical for CPOE projects.
- Make CPOE mandatory.
- Do not call it a "pilot."
- Do not withdraw CPOE go-live support too quickly.

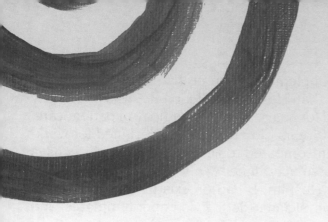

One Size Does Not Fit All: Multihospital EHR Implementation

Editor: Pam Charney

Key Words:	Project Categories:	Lessons Learned Categories:
emergency department, implementation, productivity, training, workflow	inpatient electronic health record (EHR), computerized provider order entry (CPOE)	implementation approaches, staffing resources, training, workflow

 Case Study

A multihospital health system opened a brand new hospital (Hospital A) with a strong focus on a paperless system by using cutting-edge technology and innovation. An electronic health record (EHR) vendor was selected to assist with this goal. While a few minor issues were identified, Hospital A went into operations fairly smoothly. The Emergency Department (ED) at Hospital A used a tracking board, computerized physician order entry (CPOE), and documentation in the EHR by both nurses and physicians. Daily census in Hospital A's ED was low, and the system was used for all patients presenting to the ED. Based on this success, the health system decided to implement the system at its other hospitals.

The next hospital (Hospital B) to implement the enterprise EHR hospital-wide had much different characteristics than Hospital A. Hospital A was brand new and had been specifically designed for heavy use of technology in patient care. In contrast, Hospital B was over 50 years old and was not designed for workflows involving an EHR. Also, when compared to Hospital A, the daily census and acuity for Hospital B's ED was much higher. While Hospital A went live from the start with the new EHR, Hospital B had preexisting workflows that covered nursing documentation, physician ordering via paper templates, and the dictation of patient encounters.

There was also a difference in the IT infrastructure and training capacity between the two sites. Staff at Hospital A were given two weeks EHR training before the hospital began admitting patients. Staff at Hospital B had full-time patient responsibilities, so training was scheduled during off-duty hours. Despite this, the vendor noted that the ED nursing and physician staff of Hospital B were very engaged in the training agenda.

Unfortunately the EHR go-live at Hospital B had an enormous negative impact on ED workflow. Staffing had been increased for both nurses and physicians for go-live, but the time required for both nursing and physician documentation, along with additional time needed for CPOE, exceeded expectations. The percentage of patients who left without being seen increased to a high of 12 percent from a baseline of 2 percent resulting in lost volume and hospital revenue. It took six months to return to baseline for this metric. Additional nursing and physician hours were still required with an even greater increase in hours than initially planned during go-live. Patient satisfaction, which was steady for the previous year at the 70th percentile, dramatically dropped to the fifth percentile in the first three months following go-live before beginning to trend upwards again.

Some of the issues that accounted for this included

- A steep learning curve for documentation
- Staff documenting by typing rather than using templates due to missing options and fields on the templates
- Difficulty in finding common items and areas for documentation in the system

These issues resulted in increased time spent on documentation and less time on patient care. System inefficiency in the higher volume ED at Hospital B caused the need for additional nursing and physician staffing, leading to increased costs for the hospital and physician group.

Some of the unintended consequences also included the need for the nursing and medical directors to spend countless hours documenting system issues and engaging in rework and redesign. There were ongoing biweekly team meetings with the ED leadership, health information management, accounting, and the coding teams to improve documentation issues. Nurses and physicians were also required to complete addendums to correct charting issues identified after charts had been created. This created additional nonpatient work time for the staff.

Based on their experience at Hospital B, the health system administration decided to hold the implementation at the other system hospitals. They are reevaluating their choice of EHR vendor due to the issues inherent in the design of the current system.

 Author's Analysis

Hospital A was able to use the system due to its lower acuity and census. Even though some of the issues with the documentation were consistent between the two sites, staff had significantly different availability to work on the issues. Staff at Hospital A had sufficient time to find items in the EHR and create needed workarounds while staff at Hospital B did not have this luxury.

There are several recommendations that can be made to help correct some of the issues seen in Hospital B's implementation.

1. *Nurses and physicians need to be involved in the build and testing prior to go-live.*

   Since the system was already being used at Hospital A, there was very limited involvement of the clinical staff in the application build for Hospital B. As a result, required documentation fields were missing, resulting in significant workarounds and workflow inefficiencies. Also, since there were no Hospital B clinicians involved in the build and testing, there were fewer superusers available for support during the Hospital B implementation phase.

2. *Leverage system expertise; rotate clinical users from other go-live sites to Hospital B to experience the system in a high-volume ED.*

   Having nursing and physician staff rotate from Hospital A to Hospital B during go-live would add experienced users in the ED. Not only would this have benefited the go-live site at Hospital B, but it would have given additional experience and learning to the staff of Hospital A related to issues that might arise when Hospital A's census increased in the future.

3. *Anticipate at least a six-month impact in productivity, and the need for additional nursing and physician staffing.*

   Depending on the workflow and capacity of the ED and on the EHR vendor, there might be a significant impact on not only productivity, but also patient satisfaction. Plans and budgets might need to be adjusted to keep additional staff in order to deal with the increased demands on clinical staff by the EHR.

4. *Provide 30-day and 90-day reeducation sessions.*

During the postop live meetings to address issues, a recurrent theme of lack of follow-up vendor-sponsored training sessions was identified. Not only would additional training allow for additional interaction with the vendor, but it would also foster feedback discussions about issues with current EHR workflow.

 ## Editor's Commentary

Administrators at multifacility healthcare systems are often able to take advantage of cost savings due to their large-volume purchasing habits. It is not uncommon for large healthcare systems to require that all facilities utilize the same vendors for medications, supplies, and equipment. Requests for supplies not included on the formulary frequently necessitate detailed paperwork, several layers of approval, and other tactics. Thus, it is not surprising that administrators at the hospital system described here felt that the same EHR would be appropriate for each hospital in the system.

In this case study, decision makers for the healthcare system felt they were achieving economy of scale by using the same EHR for Hospital B. Using the same system would save enormous amounts of time and money if it were successful. However, implementation of an EHR is certainly not as simple as deciding which medications and supplies to stock. Therefore, key points that could have prevented this failure were missed.

It is not clear what (if any) discussions were had with the EHR vendor concerning differences in size and focus of the hospitals in the system. Even if the software was designed to function well regardless of facility size and patient mix, the patient care environment and staff were significantly different between the two facilities, which most likely played a significant role in the failure of the EHR implementation at Hospital B.

Training is a key component in EHR implementation. Given that Hospital A had a successful implementation following two weeks of training with no patient care responsibilities, staff at Hospital B should have received even more intensive training. While clinician resistance to use of EHRs is often cited as a roadblock to implementation, it appears that physicians and nurses at Hospital B were not resisting and were engaged and willing. However, it would be difficult at best to achieve the same level of training as that achieved by Hospital A. Given this reality, it is surprising that leadership in the system did not think to rotate some staff from Hospital A to Hospital B to provide additional support "on the ground."

Hospital A had infrastructure to support use of the EHR while Hospital B did not. Thus successes that were achieved at Hospital A in a short period of time could not be expected to occur at Hospital B because Hospital B's environment of care was not designed for EHR use. Chances are that simple ergonomic principles such as workstation placement, number of available computers, lighting, and room design were significantly different, leading to additional stress placed on providers at Hospital B.

Therefore, what was initially touted as a wildly successful EHR implementation at one hospital in a multisite system rapidly turned into an EHR failure when well-meaning administrators attempted to install the same system into a significantly different environment of care. EHR success depends on many factors; people, software, and infrastructure are key. Neglecting to address one of these factors can have significant adverse consequences.

 Lessons Learned

- Local nursing and physician involvement in EHR build and testing prior to go-live is essential.
- Anticipate clinician productivity losses and plan accordingly.
- Leverage internal expertise—rotate clinician users from one go-live site to another.
- Provide follow-up training after go-live.

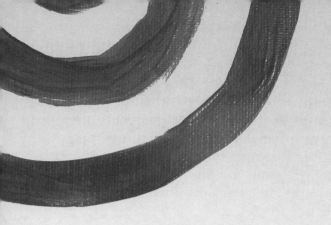

CHAPTER

3

Hospital Objectives vs. Project Timelines: An Electronic Medication Administration Record (eMAR)

Editor: Brian Gugerty

Key Words:

clinical information system, clinician leadership, help desk, medication administration, stakeholder input, workstations on wheels (WOWs)

Project Categories:

electronic medication administration record (eMAR), inpatient electronic health record (EHR)

Lessons Learned Categories:

communication, leadership/ governance, staffing resources, technology problems

 Case Study

The chief information officer (CIO) at a large teaching hospital, with support from executive management at the hospital, committed to implementing an electronic medication administration record (eMAR) with bedside documentation. The project was to be featured in the hospital's Joint Commission accreditation inspection during the next year. The CIO highlighted the risks inherent in paper MARs including the limited ability for a nurse to have up-to-date information from a patient's paper medication list.

A medicine teaching service was selected for the pilot. The hospital had already implemented broad functionality with a robust clinical information system, but the eMAR represented the first initiative that required 100 percent compliance by clinicians for clinical data entry, rather than the optional computerized provider order entry (CPOE) and clinical documentation modules, diagnostic test results system, and picture archiving and communication system (PACS) implemented previously. Several dependencies were identified during the early planning stages for the project:

- Extensive development of an integrated medication management system by the core healthcare information system (HIS) vendor, including new functionality for CPOE, pharmacy medication management, and the eMAR

- Workflow transformation for nurses, pharmacists, and physicians in the medication management process (from order entry by physicians, through order verification and medication preparation by pharmacists, to medication administration and patient assessment by nurses)

- New hardware procurement and installation to support the new eMAR, including a wireless network in the pilot inpatient unit

- Software configuration by the hospital information technology (IT) team and the vendor

- Implementation of the new software

- Training of all involved staff

The vendor worked with an interdisciplinary team of IT staff, nurses, pharmacists, and physicians to develop the functionality necessary to support best practices for medication management, from ordering to administration. Various committees met monthly, weekly, and even daily, with participants numbering from 2 to 40 depending on the topic addressed. The collective input and collaboration enabled the group to explore new concepts of interdisciplinary medication management, including pharmacy-physician communication for medication dose adjustment and confidential reporting of adverse drug events and medication errors.

Vendors demonstrated workstations on wheels (WOWs) of different sizes, weights, and with varying degrees of mobility, to the nursing and IT groups. The interdisciplinary group evaluated different laptops, recognizing that size, weight, ease of use, and even battery life would be important to the success of the eMAR. Best practices in system design and implementation appeared to be in place for the important patient safety initiative; the hospital continually stressed the importance of the project for the Joint Commission visit.

Project timelines began to slip. With only a few months before the scheduled go-live, the vendor delayed the delivery of the software. Additionally, the hospital's help desk became overburdened with support issues for existing systems, including problems of access to clinical systems, certain functions of the HIS, and properly functioning printers, computers, and monitors. In the final month before go-live, the mobile computer vendor announced a delay in the delivery of the WOWs for the pilot.

Several clinician leaders requested that the project wait until all systems could be fully tested and until the hospital refocused on routine operations after the scheduled Joint Commission visit, but the CIO remained committed to completing the initiative because it was to be a highlight in the Joint Commission visit. Ultimately, all devices arrived on the eMAR pilot medicine inpatient unit; the IT team implemented the software; and the nursing unit went live. For several days, the IT team staffed the pilot unit around the clock with nurses trained in the new eMAR to assist physicians, pharmacists, and nurses with the rollout. Clinical and administrative staff reacted well to the rollout, and the Joint Commission inspection team noted the achievement as evidence of leadership in the field of healthcare technology. Then, the focus on the pilot unit faded.

Over the next few weeks, several changes occurred on the pilot unit. The nurses who regularly staffed the unit, and whose average age was about 10 years older than those who selected the WOWs for the eMAR, complained of difficulty reading the small fonts on the screens of the WOWs. Nurses who rotated to the medicine unit after the heavily staffed rollout said they received inadequate training on the eMAR and preferred the previous paper MAR. The WOWs began crashing and freezing during regular use, requiring frequent reboots; nurses found that leaving the devices standing in the nursing station prevented such dysfunction but also prevented bedside use of the technology. Calls to the IT help desk for support went unanswered for up to 72 hours. Meanwhile, the CIO continued to discuss the successful pilot, unaware that nurses on the pilot unit had begun to print out a paper MAR for use on each shift; the paper MAR could be brought to the patient's bedside. The nurses relied on the paper MAR for patient care, updating changes in the patient's record at the end of the shift, just as they did prior to the rollout of the eMAR. During follow-up interviews at the pilot site, the nurses on the unit were surprised to learn that corporate management at the health system celebrated the achievement of the hospital's pilot eMAR; the nurses described the implementation as a disaster and a waste of resources. They had reverted to their original paper-based practices.

Author's Analysis

This failed implementation highlights many lessons about HIT initiatives, including failed project planning, failed technology configuration and testing, and failed leadership. Most importantly, clinical IT initiatives require the leadership of the clinician end-users. If the nursing department had led or co-led the eMAR initiative, the ensuing problems would have been less likely to develop unmonitored; as the nurses discovered problems with software, hardware, or training, the nursing department would have had the authority to slow, modify, or halt the initiative, instead of remaining unaware of the issue. If the project team had not faced an arbitrary deadline, such as a Joint Commission visit, but rather focused on completing the implementation successfully, adequate time might have allowed the discovery of the inadequate wireless network and staff training. Also, the experience underscores the role of the IT help desk during implementation and support of information systems. Help desks and IT support must create support processes sufficient for the applications and environments in hospitals, which include immediate response to problems in acute care areas. Often, the cost and staff of an enlarged help desk is not included as part of a system rollout, which can lead to support shortfalls after go-live. As a tool, IT offers opportunities to transform healthcare in an unprecedented manner; however, a CIO must strategize to work within the given resources of a health system or to expand those resources as required for expanding initiatives. In the case of the failed eMAR, a technology strategy outpaced the operating plan of a hospital as well as the capacity of an IT department. The resulting failure cost money, staff efficiency, and possibly compromised clinical care.

 ## Editor's Commentary

The eMAR pilot project described in this case study was ambitious from the outset. Its success depended on software to be developed by the software vendor, workflow changes across clinical departments, and a host of new hardware from WOWs to wireless networks. Also, there was a lot riding on the success of the pilot because it was a showcase for the medical center for the Joint Commission visit. An experienced project manager would have sized up this project from the very beginning as one with an inordinately high degree of risk of failure emanating from multiple sources. Hindsight is, relatively speaking, easy, however.

Yet despite the "could have been predicted" software and hardware delays and the "should have been anticipated" help desk degradation all occurring prior to go-live (go-live is usually defined as the one- to four-week period after the system is turned on), they pulled it off! The pilot go-live was a success. Then, a classic occurrence happened. The powers that be declared victory, moved on to other things, and withdrew resources. Research has demonstrated three phases to healthcare IT projects: preimplementation, go-live, and postimplementation. All three phases should be optimally managed so that project objectives stand a chance of being achieved and the gains from the new processes and technology solidify, thus becoming the new norm for the clinical environment. Then and only then can closure truly occur.

It appears that this project had some serious faults in the preimplementation period, including poor project planning, failed technical configuration, and near absence of testing, as the author pointed out in the discussion on lessons learned. Despite these shortcomings, the pilot could have been salvaged if the focus and resources showered on the project during go-live remained, even in an attenuated form, during the postimplementation period. All the issues mentioned as real problems appeared after the system was turned on and especially after the extra support during go-live was withdrawn: small font sizes; inadequate training of nurses floating to the pilot unit; crashing WOWs; and near total collapse of the help desk. Taken individually with merely adequate resources and proper management focus, these issues could have been easily resolved. Adequate and proper attention during the postimplementation period would likely have resulted in the planned new workflows, which the author did not state were problematic and therefore were presumably acceptable, solidifying the patient safety improvements being truly actualized. Some project managers and IT/clinical informatics staff treat such a new application in just this way for a pilot, providing adequate or even light preimplementation planning, showering the go-live phase with support, and addressing problems in the postimplementation period. When most of the issues are resoloved on the pilot unit, where they should be expected to occur, then and only then is the application rolled out to other units.

I could not agree more with the author's statement that "most importantly, clinical IT initiatives require the leadership of the clinician end-users" if by leadership it is understood that the clinician end-user literally has to lead the project. Perhaps the widely used (outside of the US, anyway) PRINCE2 project management methodology (PRINCE2 2013) where the project manager reports to a project board composed of an executive sponsor from the organization, a senior representative of the end-user community, and a senior technical representative throughout the entire project, could allow effective clinical end-user leadership. The glaring leadership failure in this case study, in my mind at least, was with the CIO focusing on the achievement of his or her apparent real goal of creating "evidence of leadership in the field of healthcare technology" at the expense of solidifying carefully crafted new processes that improved patient safety.

 Lessons Learned

- Clinician leadership is critical to HIT initiatives.
- IT support is critical during, and just after, a go-live.
- Effective project planning includes proper resource management.

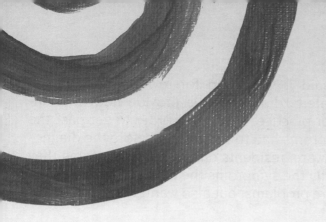

CHAPTER 4

Clinical Quality Improvement or Administrative Oversight: Clinical Decision Support Systems

Editor: Jonathan Leviss

Key Words:	Project Categories:	Lessons Learned Categories:
clinical decision support, clinical guidelines, data quality, quality assurance, workflow	computerized provider order entry (CPOE), inpatient electronic health record (EHR)	communication, workflow

 ## Case Study

Hospital administration was proud because clinicians at their small hospital were using a new clinical decision support system that alerted them when standard clinical practices were not followed. The system checked laboratory and medication orders against diagnoses in one specialty area, matched those diagnoses with symptoms for conditions, and also issued alerts when various data indicated abnormalities. The new system, the administration was convinced, was improving quality. It worked so well that they wanted to extend its use from inpatient to ambulatory care.

Direct observations and questions of end-users raised additional questions, however. Some attending physicians said the system was good, but was mainly for less skilled clinicians or for residents who still needed to learn.

Those residents and clinicians said it was good for reviewing diagnostic criteria and guidelines, but the alerts did not really provide new information or result in changed orders or practice. Further, in order to get past the requirement that all required symptoms had to be entered before the diagnosis would be accepted by the software, residents entered the symptoms they knew to be required, not necessarily the symptoms the patient had. The head of resident training knew there were problems, but also wanted to support the administration.

The administration had tried to do everything right. They used a participatory design approach and the head of quality assurance, himself a physician, was a key figure in the project. A local computer scientist had produced the system in close consultation with clinical and quality assurance staff. All clinicians were trained to use the system, as were residents when they began their rotations at this hospital.

Clinical staff, however, did not feel involved in creating the system or in determining when and how it was used. Clinicians saw the system as the administration's reporting tool, whereas the administration described the system as benefiting clinicians and improving clinical care. Further, the clinical staff felt pressured, as they had recently gone through a merger with a nearby hospital and were adjusting to new ways of doing things. For them, the clinical decision support system was yet another burden.

Even with the problems, the system did report mismatches between symptoms and diagnosis, and diagnosis and orders for medications or laboratory work; it also alerted users to abnormalities. The use of this system was well in advance of other hospitals, and the administration was proud of the progress made. They did not know about the underlying issues, but had wisely brought in others to investigate before rolling out the system for outpatient care. Administration and the clinicians had different notions of success.

 ## Author's Analysis

Lesson 1: Watch what people do rather than depending only on what they say. The ways residents were gaming the system were not apparent until outside consultants observed residents showing each other how to enter data from a new patient into the system, explaining ways to circumvent some of the system's controls. Of course, it was not presented quite that starkly, but almost.

Lesson 2: Pay attention to data quality and to influencing factors. Quality assurance was based on the data entered by the clinicians. Quality assurance staff thought that data entered by clinicians improved care, as documented by reports derived from these data. Clinicians, though, were sometimes entering data that reflected their understanding of system requirements rather than their examination of the patient, even when they knew the two might be in conflict. Consider trustworthiness of data in light of system requirements and reward structures.

Lesson 3: Incorporation of practice guidelines into clinical decision support systems does not necessarily result in increased compliance with the guidelines if workarounds and "system gaming" occur.

Lesson 4: There always will be problems. The trick is to identify the problems before they cause harm. Evaluation is necessary and should be done in skillful and nonthreatening ways that can uncover what is happening on the floors, in treatment areas, in residents' rooms—anywhere HIT is used, or supposed to be used. Often evaluation needs to be independent—either independent from the project team or the health system.

 ## Editor's Commentary

The case study highlights three key lessons: integrating effective clinical decision support is challenging; clinicians are people—they work in health systems and are affected by the current issues and culture of their organization; and projects require effective ongoing evaluation.

The wealth of literature on failed and successful computerized decision support documents the difficulties in introducing the right knowledge to physicians at the right point in care delivery without creating burdensome work or providing information that is already known or irrelevant to a particular patient. Additional references discussing this topic are included in the Suggested Readings section of Appendix C (Killelea et al. 2007; Kuperman et al. 2007; Kuperman et al. 2006).

Introducing information systems to clinical care requires changing the way clinicians interact with patients and gather and process information and challenges their decision-making at the point of care in front of both colleagues and patients. These changes can be stressful for clinicians; if other major stressors already exist, such as a recent hospital merger, new programs to measure clinicians' quality performance, or decreased physician income, then the stress of a new HIT system may be impossible to bear. Organizations need to recognize the stress level and tolerance for change of their own staffs and plan accordingly so that successful initiatives can be introduced at appropriate times. A delayed project that succeeds is more valuable, and less expensive, than a project started on time that fails.

Objective evaluation is critical to determine what aspects of a project should be continued, or expanded, and what aspects should be modified.

Depending on the size of the project, scope, and complexity, an evaluation could be extensive or brief. Part of ongoing evaluation also requires regular, open communication between the end-user community, the health system management, and the IT project team. Most health systems that succeed in creating the open dialogue between these groups have a system of interdisciplinary informatics governance—models range from interdisciplinary committees to role-based committees with committee chairs joining together in interdisciplinary forums to foster open communication. Both approaches typically involve quality management. The essential component is the opportunity for hospital management, IT, and the clinicians to express their views, concerns, and experiences, while also listening to those of the other groups. Transparent discussions about positive and negative aspects of HIT initiatives help reveal problems early for effective resolution. Sometimes, outside expertise is required to objectively evaluate a project and to remove any positive or negative bias; "outside" could mean simply someone other than the project team members or a contracted consultant with expertise in the area of the project for evaluation. Large health systems could even rotate individuals to facilities other than their primary site of work to serve as evaluators. Evaluation should be part of the improvement cycle (and ideally the entire project life cycle) of an HIT project, as it provides insight that can further improve the initiative.

 Lessons Learned

- Expect problems; the key is evaluating projects to identify problems and address them early.

- IT quality assurance requires some in-depth review of data, clinician workflow, and other details of a new process and/or technology.

- Organizational culture and current circumstances may limit the ability of members to change processes. A culture that inhibits direct and open communication leads to diminished stakeholder input in favor of conflict avoidance behaviors that often defeat the intent of HIT systems.

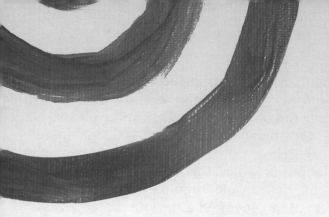

Disruptive Workflow Disrupts the Rollout: Electronic Medication Reconciliation

Editor: Gail Keenan

Key Words:	Project Categories:	Lessons Learned Categories:
CMIO, CPOE, EHR, meaningful use, medication reconciliation, pharmacist, workflow	inpatient electronic health record (EHR), computerized provider order entry (CPOE), electronic medication administration record (eMAR), pharmacy IS	implementation approaches, leadership/ governance, system design, workflow

 Case Study

After several years of a poorly focused information technology (IT) effort, a four-hospital health system created a new health informatics department and hired a chief medical information officer (CMIO) in 2006. The IT direction changed dramatically thereafter, as the organization entered into partnership with a single electronic health record (EHR) vendor. Between 2006 and 2011, the health system implemented nursing documentation, electronic medication administration record (eMAR), bar code medication administration (BCMA), longitudinal allergies and medication histories, and computerized physician order entry (CPOE) at all four hospitals. After having received systemwide approval in 2010, the health system moved quickly in 2011 to add a fully electronic medication reconciliation program into its EHR as a means of meeting American Recovery and Reinvestment Act (ARRA) of 2009 Meaningful Use requirements.

The new medication reconciliation program was quite different from the existing system in that it was fully electronic, required a pharmacist to interview each patient on admission, and generated a new discharge report. In the existing medication reconciliation system a clinician (nurse, physician, or pharmacist) entered all patient allergies and home medications into a longitudinal component of the EHR. Once gathered in the EHR, this data supported the generation of a paper report that was used to complete the medication reconciliation process. Providers liked the process because it was easy to complete, often taking as little as five seconds for reconciling a complex patient medication list. Clinicians also acknowledged its value and ease of use in making decisions about which medications to continue and discontinue at each transition of care (such as admission, transfer level of care, and discharge). The use of pharmacists to carry out the major portion of the medication reconciliation in the new system would involve a major workflow change necessitating hiring of additional pharmacists.

The leaders of the organization were nonetheless very supportive of the new system, believing that assigning the pharmacist a primary role in medication reconciliation was an excellent strategy for improving medication outcome. In fact, the enthusiasm for the new system was so high that the purchasing committee and hospital executive were willing to waive a small pilot because of the need to turn on the system in all four hospitals at the same time. As a result the impact to workflow was never fully assessed prior to purchase and implementation of the new system. Go-live thus commenced without a clear understanding of how the system would affect workflow. Once live, however, it was quickly learned that the entry and reconciliation of complex medication lists was taking most pharmacists more than 30 minutes. Even the most savvy EHR pharmacists required at least 20 minutes to complete complex reconciliations. Two weeks after go-live at all hospitals, workflow delays and provider dissatisfaction became problematic and the CMIO and hospital executives made a decision to discontinue the use of the new medication reconciliation program.

 ## Author's Analysis

There were a number of points of failure that resulted from the lack of attention to important details. The health system did not and should have considered the following prior to implementation:

- Set an acceptable time for completing electronic medication reconciliation for each transition of care (such as admit, transfer, and discharge) and validate that the time frame is achievable in the new system.

- Determine which tasks could be done simultaneously and which tasks should be supported by the new electronic system (such as discontinuing meds when transferring level of care, or continuing a number of medications upon discharge).

- Identify provider "mindsets" that could not be corrected by electronic medication reconciliation systems (such as providers who refused to take more than five seconds in the process and instead placed a vertical line through the continue columns for all medications (an unsafe practice).

- Assess vendor standard reports for relevance to one's own organization; anticipate the need for customization, including the impact of customization on the project resources and timeline.

- Provide critical and concrete evidence that the new system will work as expected before full implementation (such as bypassing a pilot because of the requirement that the system be "turned on" everywhere all at once to later learn that it was possible to hide the new system while piloting it).

 ## Editor's Commentary

EHRs and their components are extremely complex and require systematic and careful evaluation before purchase and implementation in practice. There are countless examples of very expensive systems being bought and implemented and failing miserably due to poor evaluation up front. As a result, not only are the initial expenses of the system lost (in those situations where the system is scrapped) but additional expenses are incurred, frequently much higher than the original costs, to reconcile problems that result. As such, there is no better strategy for containing the cost of EHRs than doing one's homework ahead of purchase and implementation. The interesting aspect of this case is that there were knowledgeable people involved in the decisions but they clearly did not do their homework and suffered "expensive" consequences.

One wonders why organizations fail to do their homework when making expensive decisions given the devastating financial outcomes that can occur. In some instances the parties to the decision do not have sufficient knowledge to make the right decision, while in others wishful thinking seems to be the culprit. Either way there should be no excuse allowed for failure to systematically evaluate the impact of a costly product given the potential negative financial and other outcomes that can occur for the organization and healthcare in general. The fact of the matter is that it is sometimes hard to measure the impact of EHR-related decisions and accountability for them. When accountability is not clearly specified, there is no incentive to ensure the best decisions are made. In this case one could blame the purchasing committee, the CMIO, or the key administrators involved in the decision. In the end, however, when the accountability is diffused, there is no real accountability.

To limit or avoid negative outcomes for major EHR-related purchases, it is absolutely essential that there be a process that is routinely followed and a mechanism of accountability. The rush to put in a new EHR or add new components to existing ones to meet the Office of the National Coordinator for Health Information Technology's (ONC's) Meaningful Use criteria is certain to be facilitating decision-making that is less than thorough. The shortsightedness of poorly evaluated decisions may bring the Meaningful Use incentives to an organization but ultimately create the need for costly downstream fixes to poor solutions. Had the organization in this case used a systematic process in its evaluation of the new medication reconciliation system they would have uncovered many of the problems that were discovered after implementation. The excitement over the new model and the desire to capture Meaningful Use incentives caused this organization to invoke "wishful" thinking in their actions. If an organization requires the use of a standard policy for evaluating major EHR procurements wishful thinking decisions can be avoided. Such a policy would include both the steps for systematic evaluation of EHR products and a clear mechanism of accountability. The mechanism for accountability, for example, might be to have all members of the purchasing committee sign a letter indicating that the evaluation process produced clear and compelling evidence that the product will work as intended in the organization with no additional costs.

 ## Lessons Learned

- The impact of new electronic systems on provider workflow must be assessed prior to full implementation in order to avoid unintended consequences.

- Standard features of proposed products must be evaluated in order to ensure that the new features work within an organization.

- A standard evaluation process and lines of accountability must be created for decisions related to major EHR products in order to eliminate "wishful decision making."
- Never assume anything about an EHR product and application of it to an organization in the absence of convincing evidence.

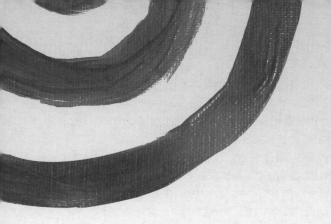

CHAPTER 6

Anatomy of a Preventable Mistake: Unrecognized Workflow Change in Medication Management

Editor: Jonathan Leviss

Key Words:	Project Categories:	Lessons Learned Categories:
adverse drug event, CPOE, EHR, medication administration, nursing, pharmacy, workflow	inpatient electronic health record (EHR), computerized provider order entry (CPOE), electronic medication administration record (eMAR), pharmacy IS	implementation approaches, leadership/governance, system design, workflow

 ## Case Study

A hospital-wide electronic health record (EHR) was installed in a midsized community hospital. This was the first installation of the product within the healthcare system. There were three other systems in use in specialty areas (Labor and Delivery, Emergency Department, and Operating Room), in addition to the lab and Picture Archiving and Communication System (PACS). The underlying structure of this EHR was such that all work was considered an individual "action" or task. Nursing staff were told that all tasks must be completed. Completion might include a documented reason for inaction. Some tasks involved multiple parts, such as administering a medication that required more than one step.

The EHR had been live for a year, and although many issues had been addressed, some were still outstanding. Medical records remained in a hybrid format, electronic or paper. However, physician orders remained strictly on paper. Bar code medication administration (BCMA) was added nine months after the EHR was implemented. The pharmacy created a "catch-up" schedule (or forced schedule) so that all medications would be given at standard times unless otherwise ordered.

A patient was admitted to the hospital for administration of chemotherapy. During the hospitalization, the patient complained of chest pain and was found to have a high probability of pulmonary embolism on a ventilation/perfusion (V/Q) scan. At approximately 10:00 a.m., an order was written for a dose of low molecular weight heparin (LMWH) to be given every 12 hours. The order was processed at 1:00 p.m. and a dose was given by a nurse sometime shortly before going off shift at 3:00 p.m. The pharmacy had previously entered the order with a forced dosing schedule of 5:00 p.m. and 5:00 a.m. The next shift's nurse gave the regularly scheduled dose according to the routine schedule at 5:00 p.m. It was unclear what signout occurred between the nurses (they should have been using a Situation-Background-Assessment-Response [SBAR] format). The subsequent dose was given at 5:00 a.m. as scheduled. At approximately 8:00 a.m., the patient complained of being weak on standing and was found to have a massive gastrointestinal (GI) bleed, which persisted over 24 hours. Esophagogastroduodenoscopy (EGD) revealed much blood but no clear treatable source. Angiography showed a bleeding esophageal vessel that was successfully embolized.

The case was reviewed utilizing a root cause analysis (RCA) methodology. Difficulty accessing the pertinent information in the EHR confounded the analysis. Key findings included the following issues:

- Inability of the nursing staff to see the entire day's medication schedule at once

- Inadequate handoff between nursing staff members

- Inclusion of high-risk/high-alert medications in the forced schedule process

Nursing staff were never provided a screen equivalent to the paper medication administration record (MAR), although one had been created for physician use after complaints were received. Instead, nurses needed to check multiple screens to find when the last dose was actually administered. In fact, medications were not seen in relation to any other medication or dosing regimen.

Actions taken after the RCA included the following steps:

- Exclusion of LWMH from forced schedule
- Creation of an alert prompt to remind nurses to check "last dose administered" for high-risk/high-alert medications
- Education of nursing staff about contacting pharmacy to reset the forced schedule if a medication was given late
- Retraining of nursing staff for SBAR use at shift change
- Addition of an alert (via BCMA) to the pharmacy
- Creation of a full MAR screen for nursing use

 ## Author's Analysis

The specific situation in this case is unfortunately not unusual. Workflow changes are common, and even expected, with implementation of EHRs. Many problems occur because evaluations of the preexisting workflows are either not done at all or overlooked. At times, potential areas for new errors may not be easily identified without a skilled and thorough workflow evaluation. Assessment of the future state workflow should have identified potential risks and points of failure for the new medication system.

This error occurred one year after the system was fully implemented. It is unknown if there were any similar overdoses that did not lead to patient harm between the initial go-live date and the date of this event. The continuous process of monitoring and addressing problems should not have ended just because the technology was live.

Task management within this product is poorly designed, as both pharmacy and nursing staff members need to go through multiple screens to administer each medication (even with BCMA), and charting when a drug is not given (held for any reason or skipped due to timing issues) is even more difficult (five screens and an average of five minutes). What appear to be straightforward orders (such as discontinue Foley cath) involve multiple related tasks that are not linked, thus requiring the nurse to select the task to discontinue (such as discontinue Foley) and also the associated care task (such as discontinue Foley care); these two items are in totally different areas of the documentation. Care processes that involve high risk require extra attention, whether the processes are paper-based or technology-enabled; the higher the risk and the greater the workflow change, the greater the need for extra attention. This need was not addressed. If the clinician end-users had been involved in the decisions and processes to select, implement, and use the technology, these shortcomings could have been identified before the project failure.

The administration is determined to make this EHR work, having already spent a significant amount of time, effort, and money (rumored to be approximately $60 million) on implementation to date. Physicians are frequently frustrated with the apparent lack of response or slow response to their complaints. Nursing staff either love the system or hate the system. (Of note, age is not a predictor of nursing staff acceptance of the system.)

Prior to this event, the company chief executive officer (CEO), chief technology officer (CTO), and chief marketing officer (CMO) met with concerned physicians about the ongoing problems that had been noted. The CEO indicated that "all development stopped" in order to meet the Meaningful Use requirements and become a Certified HIT Product so that customers could use the software to achieve Meaningful Use accreditation from the Office of the National Coordinator for HIT (ONC).

The proposed solution(s) are helpful, but it is unclear how the information about the drug dosing gets into the electronic SBAR. Adding yet another alert contributes to alert fatigue. Unless the medication can be administered through the full MAR screen, it only creates another place the nurses need to look for information. Asking busy nurses to call busy pharmacists to tell them a dose was given late is unlikely to happen on a regular basis.

 ## Editor's Commentary

The beginning of this case gives the impression that within one year of the implementation of the EHR and medication administration system, there was insufficient attention and effort on continued improvement of both the technology and how clinicians used the technology. What processes were in place to continually solicit feedback from providers about problems with the EHR? Who was the visible executive to lead this process? Was there a single clinician (or technology) lead for the EHR, who should have recognized that just as the physicians required a different view of the medication record, so might the nurses?

The typical HIT initiative is iterative, with continued attention required to enable continued improvement, similar to complex healthcare processes in general. Most health systems with CPOE and BCMA are still early in their own experiences and learning how to best use and optimize these technologies. Extra vigilance for detected and potential problems is critical, with an effective improvement cycle to address problems. Executive and project leaders need to transition the implementation charge of "let's use the system" to the optimization charge of "let's address the problems you are having with the system."

When the BCMA system introduced new workflows for nurses, including the "catch-up schedule" for medication, what workflow analyses did the clinical and IT teams perform? Did they perform formal failure mode and effects analysis (FMEA)? FMEA is critical to ensure the safety of new processes and technologies in healthcare. FMEA is a means of identifying and evaluating what can go wrong in a process, without requiring the experience of a negative occurrence, so that adverse events can be averted proactively. If an interdisciplinary team had evaluated the "catch-up schedule" for medication and the new medication user interface (UI) with an FMEA approach, overdosing of medications, specifically high-alert medications like anticoagulants, could have been identified as a risk and addressed (ISMP 2007). Finally, the author describes several technical shortcomings of the EHR—did the clinicians feel the benefits outweighed the problems (or vice versa)? How was this issue discussed and addressed by the health system? Often, resource constraints limit the ability to meet clinician requests for new HIT; specific technology options, vendor configuration services, or training may be determined to be too expensive or unnecessary. Why did the EHR leadership address the physicians' need for a better medication list view but not the nurses' similar need? Was the project leadership aware of the challenges for nurses reviewing a patient's medications in the new system? Was the problem identified but not addressed? Were nurses involved in system selection, workflow redesign, and implementation?

Learning from the example here, a nurse's ability to easily review patient medications is as important as a physician's; clinicians' concerns about workflow with HIT should be evaluated carefully as part of system selection, implementation, and optimization.

 Lessons Learned

- Assessing future state workflows is critical.
- High-risk care processes require extra attention.
- Targeted clinicians must be involved in decisions to select, implement, and use HIT.
- HIT projects are ongoing—once a technology is live, continuous process improvements are still needed.

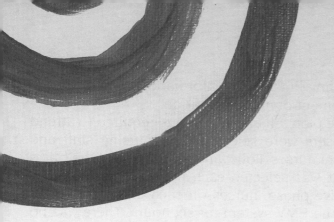

Failure to Plan, Failure to Rollout: Bar Code Medication Verification Failure

Editor: Pam Charney

Key Words:	Project Categories:	Lessons Learned Categories:
bar code, help desk, medication verification, nursing, pharmacy, workstation on wheels	inpatient electronic health record (EHR), electronic medication administration record (eMAR), pharmacy IS	implementation approaches, leadership/governance, staffing resources, technology problems, workflow

 Case Study

A community hospital implemented a bar code medication verification (BMV) system to improve tracking of medications and support safe medication administration. In addition to the software for BMV, hospital administrators purchased laptop computers stationed atop wheeled carts, or workstations on wheels (WOWs), and medication bar code scanners.

Software was selected for the program because it had the same look and feel of software currently in use to enter orders, review consults, and retrieve lab results. Two pharmacists were trained to customize the system. Additionally, two nurse managers were assigned to assist in development and implementation. Because of staffing limitations, information technology (IT) was not involved in BMV development or implementation.

BMV went live using a stepwise plan. All end-users were required to attend one classroom session. Superusers were selected from nursing staff and received the same training as other nurses. Following completion of the classroom sessions, one nursing unit was selected each month for a three-day go-live process. During the go-live phase, nurses on each unit were paired one-to-one with a superuser of the BMV system for six hours. There was no training or help desk assistance provided for use of the WOWs.

Shortly after implementation many of the laptops began to crash when the BMV system was opened. Because IT was not involved in the BMV program implementation, users were told to contact the pharmacy for assistance. Superusers were also tasked with troubleshooting hardware problems, which left little time for assisting with BMV implementation or their own nursing duties.

Facilities engineering was not involved in the program and had not been assigned to maintain or repair the laptop carts. Lacking proper authorization, they refused to assist in repairs until documentation was prepared and approved. It was not unusual to see one of the BMV pharmacist programmers roaming the floors, screwdriver in hand, repairing laptop carts.

At the end of the first year, expensive external extra-long-lasting laptop batteries with wall-mounted chargers stopped recharging so more had to be purchased. Other hardware problems were encountered. Scanner cords broke because they were not long enough and busy nursing staff had stretched them past their limit. Batteries on cordless scanners would not recharge and had to be replaced. At this point IT took on responsibility for hardware issues and during the second year of the program was able to purchase enough spare laptop batteries and scanners to service the hospital.

The IT department was able to hire more staff and was finally able to provide help desk services for the BMV program. Because of the huge backlog of work, WOWs with repair tickets would sit in unit storage rooms for days to weeks. Unit nurses felt that little or no importance was placed on how the nurses would function when the WOWs were not functional. Lacking support, nurses felt that it was assumed they would share the remaining WOWs. Former superuser nurses were occasionally able to solve some of the problems and created workarounds to keep the WOWs functional as much as possible.

When computer-savvy nurses were able to take on some repairs without authorization from IT, conflicts developed between nursing and IT. Nursing's requirements for functional WOWs for the BMV system needed to take precedence over IT support for other hospital functions, creating stress on IT staff.

As hardware and software failures increased, nurses stopped scanning medication because there were not enough scanners, laptops, or WOWs available. Workarounds were created by carrying extra ID bracelets to scan and by hand-typing drug numbers into documentation fields, which initially was only to be done for the rare case when the bar code would not scan. In this manner, nurses could sign out their medications while still sitting at the nurses' station. Medication errors were made, the same medication errors the BMV system was supposed to correct.

Medications were kept in a med room that housed a dispensing machine. Nurses had to enter their username and personal identification number (PIN) (or fingerprint), choose the patient, choose the medication, remove it, and sign out. Only a brief orientation session to this system was provided including the safety and security features of medication dispensing systems. It was not uncommon for a nurse to remove second doses of meds from the dispenser and place them in their pocket so they would not have to return to the machine for a drug they knew they would be giving in three to four hours. Although against policy, nurses routinely did this with controlled medications because in the paper system if a nurse forgot to sign off the medicine, someone could sign and cosign it so the record was kept properly. However, the signature omission would be maintained in the new BMV system and the pharmacy department would note the discrepancies in the count of the meds: two doses removed from the dispenser, only one dose recorded. Medications went missing. Lastly, password sharing was not uncommon as most nurses failed to realize the implications and gravity of this practice.

 ## Author's Analysis

Within two years of go-live, the system was considered a failure; the lack of support from IT and facilities engineering was seen as the primary cause of the failure. Ultimately, the entire EHR system was abandoned for a newer platform that integrated CPOE, test results, and all clinical notes including physician and ancillary departments. Several wrong strategies led to this failed effort. The project lacked clear collaborative partnership between nursing and IT. While clinical leadership is critical to a health IT initiative, so is IT leadership. The clinical leadership contributed content and strategic leadership, but that is not sufficient for success. The lack of involvement of the hospital's IT department meant that critical project resources were absent from the planning stages through implementation and into the support stage. Engineering's input into device selection might have averted the hardware complications that occurred, such as the problems with batteries, computer carts, and scanners. A knowledgeable help desk would have been able to support the clinician users who struggled with a technology that was critical to patient care.

The hospital ultimately developed a different approach to EHR adoption. Computer training courses are available for all employees as one step in preparing staff. In general, the hospital leadership has higher hopes that the new federal and state regulations and incentives as well as a more integrated approach will ease the burden for all staff.

 ## Editor's Commentary

Bar code medication verification programs are sophisticated, complex systems that are supposed to increase the safety of patients and decrease errors in medication administration. It is imperative that all departments of a healthcare organization be involved from the planning stage and that they are adequately prepared to meet the inevitable challenges. Failure to properly plan, design, and implement such complex systems is quite often a guarantee that the system will fail. In this case, it is not surprising that the system failed. It is surprising, however, that the system was kept in place for two years.

Although not specifically stated, it appears individuals with IT project management expertise were not involved with this project. The first step towards system failure appears to be that system users were not included in system selection. Instead, a system was chosen that had the same look and feel of software currently in use. What is not known is how well that system was meeting user needs for medication administration. Individuals selected to lead the project were most likely not aware of end-user needs and expectations and certainly did not have the knowledge and skill needed to implement an IT project of this magnitude. A cascade of poor communication, lack of understanding of workflow, and insufficient training and support led to the eventual system failure.

It would be difficult to pinpoint one specific misstep that caused the BMV system to fail. The decision by hospital administrators to purchase equipment for the system apparently without involvement from nursing, IT, or pharmacy suggests a "top down" management style, where management dictates exactly how work is to be accomplished. Chances are that administrators did not see the need to develop and implement a project plan. There was no individual assigned overall responsibility for the system. Instead components of the system were assigned to different departments who did not communicate or collaborate with each other.

Chances are that appropriate attention to the need for strong leadership, appropriate project management, and some ability for the departments involved to collaborate and solve problems (instead of blaming each other) would have given the BMV system a fighting chance for success.

Lessons Learned

- Clinicians and IT must be included from the planning through rollout stages of complex IT projects.
- Successful implementation requires sufficient help desk staffing well beyond the go-live phase.
- Clinicians and IT need a clear understanding of each other's role and workload.
- Nursing and IT need to have a clear understanding of each other's role and workload so that conflict can be avoided.
- Engineering must participate in selection of equipment and be prepared to support hardware.

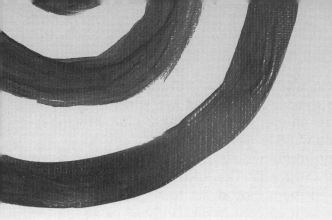

CHAPTER 8

Basic Math: HL7 Interfaces from CPOE to Pharmacy to eMAR

Editors: Larry Ozeran and Jonathan Leviss

Key Words:	Project Categories:	Lessons Learned Categories:
computerized provider order entry (CPOE), electronic medication administration record (eMAR), Health Level 7 (HL7) interface, pharmacy, test system	inpatient electronic health record (EHR), computerized provider order entry (CPOE), electronic medication administration record (eMAR), pharmacy IS	system configuration, technology problems

 Case Study

In our CPOE system, a medication order was generated for warfarin 7 mg daily. Using an HL7 interface message, the medication order was communicated to an external pharmacy system. Because there was no dispensable product of warafin 7 mg, the pharmacist converted the order into dispensable products, a 5-mg tablet and a 2-mg tablet.

Several days later, clinicians observed that the patient's anticoagulation laboratory results (INR) were at panic levels, but there had been no easily identified originating event. The anticoagulation medications were reviewed and the clinicians were surprised at the warfarin dosing – it was much higher than originally ordered. The clinicians ordered a dose of warfarin 7 mg daily, yet the order and the eMAR both indicated a dose of warfarin 14 mg. Upon review of the audit trail, the provider entered warfarin 7 mg, but after the pharmacy verification, the order was modified to warfarin 14 mg.

The first step was to implement an immediate workaround, which was to discontinue the order and reenter the medication order differently. Because the medication dose required two separate products to be dispensed (warfarin 2 mg and 5 mg), the order was reentered successfully as two separate medication orders.

 ## Authors' Analysis

The complexities of an interfaced medication order between two disparate vendor applications cannot be overestimated. Iatrogenic events can change the data outcome and affect clinical outcomes.

The complexities of HL7 include both the technology standards and the semantic standards. Events like a medication order generate an HL7 message that is communicated through an interface engine and then to the receiving system. As the message travels, each computer has the ability to interpret and even modify the content of the data based on defined algorithms.

During evaluation, the situation was replicated in our test system. The troubleshooting efforts were focused on the multiple product situation. Because the medication dose required two separate products be dispensed, the successful workaround was to enter two separate orders while the troubleshooting continued. In the CPOE system, the medication is ordered as a generic name and a dose, without product level considerations.

Appropriately, within a pharmacy application, the medication order was interpreted into the dispensing product level. Within this pharmacy system, there was functionality for a multiproduct medication order being represented as a single medication order. If the generic formulary item is the same, the medication dose requiring two products can be combined in a single order. The warfarin 7 mg order included two dispensing products—warfarin 2 mg and warfarin 5 mg.

Upon review, the original CPOE HL7 message that was sent to the pharmacy system was passed through an enterprise interface engine and then a CPOE interface engine before being received by the external pharmacy application and used the same route upon return to the CPOE system. The CPOE system identified the generic product and dose while the pharmacy system identified the generic and dispensing products required to provide the dose.

In HL7, the "RXE" segment represents the pharmacy encoded order data (Hann's On Software 2008). The "Give amount" and "Give units" values are updated during the "perfection process" (pharmacy verification). With a multiproduct order, two separate RXE segments are defined. In this case, there were two RXE segments, one for warfarin 2 mg and one for warfarin 5 mg. As the pharmacy application had a process to manage multiple RXE segments, an unexpected data transformation occurred. The result was that instead of adding the amounts to a total dose, it multiplied the subcomponents, thus generating 14 mg instead of the expected 7 mg. So the calculation was

2 RXE components × (2 mg) + 2 RXE components × (5 mg) = 14 mg

The CPOE application accepted the verification with the dose modification from the pharmacy system and changed the order view and the eMAR view of the order to a dose of 14 mg. There was no alert, only an overwriting of the original order; the modification went unnoticed until a clinical situation arose.

Once the issue was identified, additional testing confirmed the situation, and the vendor was contacted. The issue had the highest vendor priority, and a fix was available the next day. On site, reports were generated to check for any other instances of the situation, one additional patient was identified, and the clinicians were immediately involved. There were no adverse long-term impacts to either of the patients.

 Editor's Commentary

This scenario reminds us of some very important lessons.

1. *You often don't know what you don't know.*

   This is why it is critical to check all of your assumptions when something goes wrong. The authors and their institution must be commended for having a clear process for investigating problems. They planned for failure and how to manage it.

2. *Computers* **DO** *make mistakes, when we provide the wrong information or the wrong instructions.*

   There is a tendency to think that the data we get from the computer must be right, simply because it came from the computer. This expectation and the resultant complacency can blind us to embedded errors. One key component of evaluating the information exchanged by systems is thorough testing, such as that performed in a test laboratory similar to that described by the authors; rigorous testing is critical prior to implementing new technologies and even upgrades to existing systems.

What was the testing process prior to this implementation? Testing of closed loop medication systems, for example, should focus on both typical, straightforward orders as well as very complex ones, such as the warfarin order previously described. Although testing may not identify all problems, a broad testing strategy should dramatically decrease the likelihood of errors such as that described earlier. If warfarin orders were being divided automatically, perhaps other similar orders were also affected by the system, such as complex doses of medications or parenteral nutrition. Testing protocols should include these challenging scenarios. Anecdotal evidence indicates that many hospitals do not have appropriately replicated environments in which to thoroughly test systems prior to rollout; test environments may not include the full array of clinical information systems or a sufficiently large test database, or involve clinicians who understand the more sophisticated data flows that are generated during clinical care. The practice of thorough testing should be part of any technology implementation.

3. *Whenever we computerize a medical process to reduce errors, there is always a risk that new errors will be introduced.*

The currently widespread political support for CPOE and ePharmacy is appropriate, but also concerning. Many politicians see only the potential benefits and do not acknowledge or understand the potential risks. The current political and regulatory environment is setting unreasonably glowing expectations for HIT. In many ways, this specific error was caught quickly because there was an easily observable clinical effect that did not kill patients before the culprit could be identified. Had the dosing been for digoxin, a very different outcome might have resulted. In that case, it might have been very difficult to identify a pattern among a few patients because digoxin becomes toxic more slowly. We must remember that every change that can bring an improvement to our provision of healthcare can also bring new problems. We must be diligent about finding those problems. That means that managers, executives, regulators, legislators, and every other leader who plays a role in our healthcare system must be aware that technology brings costs beyond the financial, and they must support implementing technology safely. We must properly balance accuracy with rapid change.

Lessons Learned

- Perform extensive testing with a large number of scenarios involving different product level data.
- Involve clinicians who are technology savvy to participate in testing of scenarios.
- Empower all clinicians to question medication doses and other aspects of clinical care processes, even if they involve information systems.

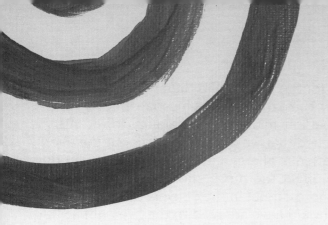

Technological Iatrogenesis from "Downtime": Pharmacy and Medication Systems

Editors: Jonathan Leviss and Larry Ozeran

Key Words:	Project Categories:	Lessons Learned Categories:
adverse event, allergy, computerized provider order entry (CPOE), downtime, medication administration, patient safety, pharmacy, training, vendor contract	inpatient electronic health record (EHR), electronic medication administration record (eMAR), pharmacy IS	communication, contracts, leadership/governance, staffing resources, technology problems, training

 Case Study

At 4 a.m. I was paged at home by the pharmacy director; I called back to hear, "one of your nurses has really messed up this time…nearly killed a patient."

I arrived at the hospital intensive care unit (ICU) break room to see a capable and experienced nurse sobbing, thinking she was solely responsible for seriously harming a patient. I felt bad—this nurse had switched from day shifts to nights to help orient several new nurses. After comforting the nurse, I listened to her recollect the events of the incident. At 2 a.m. the nurse went to the automated medication dispensing unit to obtain an antibiotic (AB) for a patient.

She selected and retrieved the AB for the patient and then promptly delivered it. Shortly after medication delivery, the patient experienced respiratory arrest.

The nurse explained that the patient had a serious allergy to the AB she administered. Immediately, I assumed that we did not know about the allergy or someone failed to enter the patient's allergy into the medication module in the pharmacy. In any case, I thought the nurse should have checked the arm band, or the chart, and been more careful in the delivery of the scheduled medications. Yes, I thought, she should have adhered to the five rights.

Later that morning, I began to complete the cumbersome paperwork that accompanies adverse events. I found the AB allergy appropriately listed in the patient's pharmacy medication profile. Next, I discovered that the nurse selected a similarly spelled, yet altogether different, medication from that ordered. The case prompted a conversation with the pharmacy director about our medication delivery system. The ICU was scheduled for the "go-live" with bar code medication administration (BCMA) in three months. I knew this situation would provide for a lively discussion at the Pharmacy and Therapeutics (P&T) Committee, as the chair believes the new technologies will help nurses stop making errors.

 ## Authors' Analysis

After conducting an investigation, followed by a root cause analysis, we found the following issues involved technology:

1. The pharmacy-unit medication cabinet interface for the ICU was inoperable, or "down," at the time of the event.

   a. The hospital required the administrator on call to be immediately notified when a system was "down."

2. The pharmacy was aware the system was down but this appeared to be a normal "update time" from 11 p.m. and 3 a.m.

   a. Paper shift reports showed that the system was down nearly 60 percent of the time during the hours of 11 p.m. and 3 a.m. (although updates were not regularly occurring).

3. The vendor acknowledged awareness that the system was down, but had not reported the issue to the P&T Committee because a fix was imminent. The vendor did not consider the system "down" because all other interfaces were functional.

4. The on-call hospitalist ordered the new medication for an unfamiliar patient in response to important new blood culture results.

a. The nurse and physician did not verbally discuss the order.

b. Follow-up testing could not duplicate the medication order in the CPOE system without an override, even with repeated mock attempts.

5. Nurses at night were used to the system being down, but day nurses rarely experienced this downtime.

a. The night nurses did not think downtime warranted an incident report.

6. The hospital had no policies and procedures to monitor technology quality, such as system reliability.

7. Most importantly, everyone thought that someone else knew about this problem.

The operational failure the nurse unexpectedly discovered was that the medication dispensing machine was unable to profile each patient's medication record. When a patient-specific medication profile was absent, the dispensing machine's entire pharmaceutical contents were readily available and the patient profile (for example, allergies) was not present as a protective layer. Notably, a clinician was able to remove the wrong medication or the wrong medication dose from the dispensing unit, an act that was only possible with an override when the pharmacy-machine interface was properly functioning. Also, the BCMA system would be rendered ineffective when the interface was disrupted, creating the precondition for potentially serious events in the other units.

HIT operational failures may result more often than reported in the literature because of stealth operational failures that only manifest when a patient is seriously harmed and investigation and root cause analysis are conducted. The sociotechnical system is quite complex, and tightly coupled, with the propensity to generate rapid error cascades that end in technological iatrogenesis. In this case, the unanticipated latent failure, "downtime," manifested as an active error and sentinel event. When technology and people become disconnected because of "downtime" associated with system interfaces, a nontrivial latent failure is immediately present and places the system at risk for failure.

HIT system implementations in hospitals pledge to make patients safer and to provide clinicians with safety supports as they work hard to provide quality care. However, the nurse involved in this event trusted the system and became dependent on the technology without realizing the potential negative consequences. The HIT provided a safety illusion. The trust placed in the vendor to work as a partner was inappropriate. Unfortunately for the patient harmed and the nurse traumatized, the vendor did not function as a partner in safety; commercial contract concerns overrode disclosures. An important lesson learned is that all management safety expectations (reporting, expected outcomes, system reliability) should be reduced to writing as part of the contract.

 Editor's Commentary

The medication error documented in this chapter illustrates key failure points that can occur in an HIT initiative, notably the following:

- *Communication*—CPOE systems, especially when integrated with pharmacy systems and medication administration systems, eliminate much of the verbal communication between physicians, nurses, pharmacists, and even laboratory technicians or ancillary staff. When HIT systems are implemented, full workflow analyses, including communication practices, should be evaluated to identify what steps are being replaced or changed and what the potential impact might be. Sometimes a valuable check existed in the paper world that might be lost with the new process that was particularly important to a specific unit, team, or organization. Just because it is common for a system to stop functioning does not mean that it is a normal condition. Complacency about the nonfunctional status quo nearly killed a patient.

- *System Performance*—Technology downtime is a critical issue in healthcare, a continuous process that runs 24/7 all year long. Scheduled "downtimes" require specific policies and processes, just as unscheduled downtimes. They should be no longer than necessary and policies should clearly outline what clinical staff is to do during those downtimes to ensure patient safety. Physicians and nurses learn to benefit from medication safety technology and shift the focus to patient management issues not protected by an information system, such as double-checking infusion rates instead of medication name spelling. When the safety support is withdrawn from the first issue, a worse situation could result. Hospitals run disaster drills, and even fire drills, but how many run HIT downtime drills to keep staff aware of downtime processes? Downtime drills keep all staff aware of their role in alerting peers and leadership to problems and the role of incident reports for HIT problems.

- *Leadership*—Leadership must define performance criteria for an HIT initiative, including the minimal technical performance metrics, and create policies and processes for technical insufficiencies. Projects must be monitored for achieving planned metrics, and policies must be monitored for adherence.

- *Staffing/Training*—It is common in our high-stress environments where time and resources are at a premium for training to be inadequate.

In this case, the nurse on duty had not been adequately trained with regard to the limitations of the system during the night shift and had not been taught what she needed to do in order to ensure patient safety. Although it is commonplace for a new hire to be trained to become familiar with a new institution, it is less common for retraining to occur when an existing employee moves to another part of a facility, or in this case, another shift. Each area should have a standard training process, even if some of it is review for those already working for the organization.

- *Contracts*—Contracts should clearly state the goals and objectives of the business relationship between a vendor and customer, but contracts are usually invoked when something goes wrong. Project vigilance and transparent communication are the most important components of a successful customer-vendor engagement, like any relationship.

Finally, the author describes an investigation process into an adverse event that should be applied through failure mode analysis before going live with an automated solution. All of these approaches require resources that not all health systems are able to commit, but perhaps they should be required to do so.

 ## Lessons Learned

- Communication is crucial among all users and stakeholders, especially when an issue or error arises.
- System performance should be monitored continually.
- Leadership is essential to maintain focus on project and system goals and objectives.
- Staffing/training must be ongoing to ensure consistency in practice and information.
- Contracts should include minimal performance expectations in a manner that is transparent and understood by all participating parties.
- Failure mode analysis is an essential step in technology implementation prior to production use.

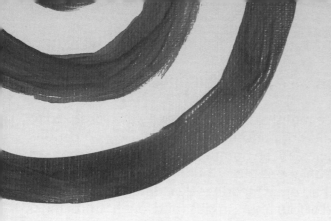

Trained as Planned: Nursing Documentation

Editor: Eric Rose

Key Words:	**Project Categories:**	**Lessons Learned Categories:**
change management, clinicians, competency assessment, electronic health record (EHR)	inpatient electronic health record (EHR)	communication, leadership/ governance, project management, staffing resources, training

 Case Study

We have all heard about the importance of user participation in selection and implementation of clinical information systems. Several years ago this was a fundamental principle used by my team to identify units to test our electronic documentation system. Each unit selected was required to have an adequate staffing level, a low turnover rate, high morale, and full commitment to test our system for the specified test period. Interested units were told up front that each would be required to choose a core set of champions to train colleagues and lead the implementation of the change. Once units were selected, champions were identified by the nurse managers and trained by the study team. After full training, the champions assisted with training the remaining staff nurses and took responsibility for assessing and ensuring the basic competency of each before go-live. A unit was not allowed to go live until all nurses were considered to be fully trained and competent.

During routine evaluations three months after go-live, we were surprised to learn that some of the nurses could not perform even the simplest functions that had been "required competencies" in the training. Also, many of the nurses reported not hearing about the change prior to attending the first mandatory training sessions even though we had open meetings describing our participation criteria. The training consisted of four hours in class and four hours of independent study, with each member required to pass a written test and return demonstration to show competency. After probing deeper, we discovered that competencies were not tracked or evaluated consistently by each unit's champions. One major discrepancy was that some champions allowed the staff nurses to report being competent rather than insisting on the required demonstration. This fueled negative feelings about the documentation system being tested that in turn affected overall satisfaction of the users. In one instance, improper use of the system by one nurse adversely affected the quality of information available to the next nurse. In the end, costly retraining was needed to put the group back on track to offset this preventable outcome.

 ## Author's Analysis

The most important lesson we learned was one we thought we already knew—training is critical to the success of a system. Doing training correctly, however, is not so simple for a variety of reasons. Hospitals are constantly undergoing change, and it is difficult to ensure that all staff have adequate knowledge and competency to carry it out because of the nature of how a hospital arranges for staffing (for example, full time, part time, resource pools, floaters, affiliate staff). Moreover, asking individuals (champions) to take responsibility for ensuring compliance of their peers' actions is problematic in the absence of an explicit mechanism for handling noncompliance. Because we wanted our units to own the change, we fostered "participation" by allowing each unit, under the direction of the manager, to tailor the training materials to fit the setting needs. Our mistake was to assume that the competency and commitment of the nurse manager and champions was sufficient to carry out the training properly.

On reflection, it is clear that the dynamic nature of the hospital environment coupled with continuous change contributes to the bending of rules to meet deadlines. This bending may be well meaning but can lead to unintended consequences. For example, in this scenario, we understood because of time constraints, champions trusted colleagues' "self-reports" of competency, rather than requiring a demonstration of it. To address this issue, we have subsequently concentrated heavily on facilitating the creation of a training plan that is both feasible and effective and providing the necessary resources to develop and implement it. Funding excellent planning is as important as the training itself.

 ## Editor's Commentary

This story about training is certainly sobering. Its teller, even at the time the story takes place, is no dilettante or neophyte in the world of complex HIT projects, but rather a seasoned professional, schooled in the formal and informal knowledge of the field. The plan was a page right out of enlightened project management, driving ownership of the project down as far to the end-users as possible. This approach is supposed to get results and "empower" users at the same time. So can we learn anything from this story, or do we just throw up our hands and declare, "The best-laid schemes of mice and men go oft astray"?

That overused quotation may itself hold the key to a lesson this story can teach us: in HIT implementations we must plan for failure. In HIT, no plan, however carefully or wisely it is crafted, allows a "set it and forget it" approach. Each project is unique and requires careful and close monitoring from its initiation, intensely at first, and less so as things appear more and more to go according to plan.

That being said, what differences in the plan, or its execution, might have produced a better outcome, or alerted the project leaders to the risk of an undesirable outcome?

One question is whether the "right" units were really selected. It is often difficult to determine what areas in an organization are ideal for testing new technology. The stated selection criteria for units to participate in the test project (adequate staffing, high morale, and so on) seem logical enough. However, one wonders whether the "full commitment to test" the system was shared by all throughout the unit. Managers may, at times, be motivated to adopt a new technology for a variety of reasons (curiosity, enthusiasm for the potential of the technology—in some cases, with exaggerated expectations as to the benefits it will bring, anticipated elevation of status as an innovator, and so on) despite a lack of readiness in their units or departments for the technology. Looking more closely at the units whose managers volunteered for this project might have called some of them into question as candidate units. Admittedly, however, in projects such as the one described here, the perception of the unit managers may be that they are extending a "favor" by their willingness to participate, and questioning their units' fitness might be politically sensitive.

Another question lies in the selection of "champions." Much has been written on the ideal characteristics of a "user champion" in complex technology deployments.

There are few data from rigorous, controlled studies on this issue. However, general consensus exists that technology skills are a lesser predictor of success as a "champion" than respect and influence among the user community. The case history does not discuss how the champions were selected, but if the champions were self-selected through a volunteer process, or hand-selected by managers based on perceived information technology knowledge, they may have faced significant barriers to success. Given the dependence of the project on direct accountability of users to the champions for demonstrating competence with the system, the champions, when faced with resistance on the part of more senior and/or politically influential colleagues among the rank-and-file users, may have felt inhibited from attempting to force the issue of demonstrating competence.

 Lessons Learned

- Continuously monitor projects for progress and desired outcomes.
- Plan training programs and provide ongoing training options for effective outcomes.
- Identify the "right" project champions.

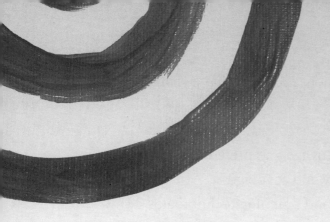

Device Selection—No Other Phase Is More Important: Mobile Nursing Devices

Editor: Gail Keenan

Key Words:	**Project Categories:**	**Lessons Learned Categories:**
mobile devices, selection process, user opinions, workflow	infrastructure and technology	leadership/governance, project management, workflow

 ## Case Study

Our story began almost two years ago. As a consultant, this author participated in a team that completed a device needs assessment for the selection of point-of-care documentation devices for Big Healthcare System (BHS). Our consultant team was engaged because of an unsatisfactory response from an employee to a member of the facility's board of directors. The question was "How did we arrive at the decision to select these certain machines that you are asking $1.7 million to purchase?"

Our team defined the following metrics for device selection:

- Device form factor analysis (workstations on wheels [WOWs], tablets, other handheld devices)

- Space availability within patient rooms during use and storage
- Provisions for spare machines
- Downtime strategies
- Analysis of various clinician usage and preferences
- Wireless networking capacity and coverage
- Integration with bar coding and scanning technologies
- Electrical outlet availability (location and quantity)
- Reallocation of existing desktop machines for physician usage

In total, this process was completed over the course of eight weeks, and upon presentation to the board of directors, our team literally received a standing ovation. Upon completion of our work, we presented our strategy and success around device selection, and the abstract of this write-up received a national award.

Based on this success, there was great confidence in our processes. In a new opportunity for a similar device selection process as part of a larger project at a Regional Community Hospital (RCH) in the West, we expected to repeat our success. The project was initiated, and RCH built a team of invested, skilled, and knowledgeable clinical and information technology staff. However, the device selection team was scheduled to meet weekly, as opposed to the concentrated "all hands on deck" efforts experienced at BHS. Thus, from the project design stage, the process was changed to be longer in duration at RCH than our process of eight weeks at BHS. Almost two years later, point-of-care devices were only just being purchased for use by nursing assistants, respiratory care therapists, and some sporadic use in the intensive care unit.

As a result of the slower, comprehensive, and methodical process for device selection, we identified opportunities that would not have been possible in a quicker, more concentrated project. Some of our notable findings are the following:

- The emergence of newer point-of-care technologies (tablets with scanners)
- Postponement of capital expenditures
- Reconciling specific challenges with wireless network coverage and capacity constraints
- Resolution of infection control issues related to device cleaning and storage
- Planning for medication administration and pharmacy delivery process changes
- Configuration of WOWs

This methodical approach created a new challenge to our credibility, especially among the nursing staff. Because significant aspects of point-of-care device selection require participation from front-line nursing staff, we engaged the nursing staff early in the selection approval process. Although early involvement provided education and buy-in, it also led to significant delays in acquisition and deployment, which caused frustration among the nursing staff.

 ## Author's Analysis

The single most important lesson learned is that the desired outcomes should dictate the decision-making process used when selecting point-of-care devices, with consideration of factors such as the necessary duration and method required. Both short and prolonged decision-making processes bring benefits and challenges. For example, the singular decisions and delays that occurred at RCH actually translated into a number of benefits. The selection team was able to develop a better understanding of the nurses' needs and to value their input, which resulted in greater buy-in among the nurses. On the other hand, the cumulative nature of the delays was a source of frustration, causing the team to appear inept and adversely influencing the senior management's perceptions of the validity of the team's recommendations. While this manuscript was being written, we neared what we hoped would be the end of the device selection and acquisition cycle. We designed a phased purchase and implementation planned to occur over the course of the next six months. This should allow for device storage, power management, and configuration as well as education, training, and workflow redesign for pharmacy and nursing staff.

Should this author participate in a similar project in the future, the experiences at both organizations will serve well. Point-of-care device selection timelines can and should be set by the interdisciplinary device selection team. While the RCH team adhered to its mission, the practical objectives were missed because of a strict interpretation.

 ## Editor's Commentary

This case study provides a great example of why it is important to fit the decision-making process to the purpose and desired outcomes of the decision and not be single-minded about the length of the timeline. Because conventional wisdom extols the merits of "decisiveness," it is no surprise that most would favor the short process of BHS in device selection if given the choice between it and the longer RCH process. Certainly the extra costs of a longer process alone provide "immediate" and powerful evidence that when presented will quickly squelch any interest in engaging in a more involved and longer selection process.

Most would agree, however, that our health technology decisions have a dramatic impact on the delivery of care and once made cannot be easily reversed. It thus is absolutely essential that the very best decisions be made in the selection phase because this is the only phase in which the purchase of a bad system can be prevented and the associated costs abated. The piece most frequently given the least attention in the selection phase is the expected impact of technology on the user, whose work should be made easier, safer, more efficient, and effective. In this scenario RCH was more cognizant of the people issues than BCH. Nonetheless, the case study did indicate that RCH lacked a rational strategy for how to incorporate the "people side" into the selection. RCH focused on learning the nurses' opinions about and getting buy-in for a system that the user had not tested under real-time conditions. Clinicians' opinions of systems that have not been fully tested under real-time conditions should not be treated as conclusive evidence of the benefits and value of the system. To remedy this repeating problem, I recommend that all organizations engage in a process by which the products being reviewed are tested under simulated conditions in a clinical setting. In this way, organizations will discover the overt and covert impact of these devices on the users and the system at large.

 ## Lessons Learned

- Structure a decision-making process to achieve the desired outcomes and communicate this to participants.

- The "selection" phase is the critical phase to prevent the purchase of bad technology; invest time and money to be very thoughtful about HIT selection.

- The opinions of users about products they have never used under real-time conditions are not solid evidence of the value of an information technology device.

- Simulate the impact of devices during evaluation under real-time conditions to better understand the effect on users and the care delivery system as a whole.

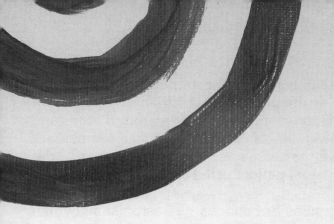

Collaboration Is Essential: Care Planning and Documentation

Editor: Jonathan Leviss

Key Words:	Project Categories:	Lessons Learned Categories:
care planning, documentation, EHR, executive management, nursing	inpatient electronic health record (EHR)	leadership/governance, system design, workflow

 ## Case Study

Several years ago, a group of researchers conducted a two-year test of an electronic care planning and documentation tool under real-time conditions in four different hospitals. The application was web-deployed and, though not directly connected to each organization's electronic health record (EHR) during the study, it appeared seamless to users. Links to the patient's EHR and the care plan application were readily accessible through tabs located on the central computer screen, enabling the effective workflow. Moreover, since the care plan information was not redundant to or directly dependent on items in the EHR it was not necessary to build a complicated interface between the two. Patient demographic information was the only redundancy and was entered separately into the care planning system on first admission to avoid creating separate HL7 admission/discharge/transfer (ADT) feeds from each test site's EHR before full testing was completed. Prior to using the application, each staff nurse at the pilot sites was trained to represent patient problems, outcomes, and interventions with standardized terms and measures and to keep the patient's plans of care current. Once competency in the application was established, the nurse was required to enter an initial care plan or update at handoff on every patient cared for by the nurse during the previous shift.

Compliance for updating care plans at handoffs was astonishingly high (80 to 90 percent) across all participant units in comparison to the less than 50 percent rate that others have found when care plan updating requirements are less stringent (such as every 24 hours) (Keenen et al. 2012). The simplicity of the system and requirement for regular updating at handoff helped ensure care plans were current and in turn supported nurses in maintaining a shared understanding of the overall care and progress toward desired outcomes, a feature lacking in contemporary EHRs. At the end of the study, the nurses in all units were significantly more satisfied with the new tool than with the previous care planning systems and advocated strongly for retention of the tool. The data collected with the system provided a rich source for examining the impact of nursing care on patient outcomes because the data were coded with standardized terminologies and stored in a carefully designed relational database. Since the typical formats of nursing documentation do not allow for meaningful evaluation of the impact of nursing care, the ability to conduct such evaluation was considered a truly transformational benefit. Finally, word about the care planning system spread to nurses in other health systems; they became interested in adopting the care planning system as well.

Unfortunately, intense advocacy by managerial and staff nurses for adopting the care planning system after the study was met with opposition from central decision makers responsible for the information technology decisions at the same hospitals. The nurses consistently were told that it was necessary to adopt a single fully integrated EHR and were assured that the EHR (either in place or to be implemented) would provide functionality similar to the care planning system. As a result, the fully tested care planning system was pulled from each of the four test organizations. Previously interested health systems and hospitals not in the study also decided not to adopt the new system for the same reasons. Ultimately the nurses in both the study and nonstudy hospitals seeking to implement the care planning and documentation system accepted the decisions of the information technology teams at their respective hospitals, trusting that the functionality would soon appear in their EHRs.

Author's Analysis

Five years later, none of the major EHR systems in the healthcare organizations described above contained the robust features of the fully tested care planning system. The care planning features of these EHR systems provide only minimal functionality that has to be tailored to meet each hospital unit's needs. As a result, the current care planning tools at these hospitals offer no improvements over the traditional systems previously in place or the proven benefits of the care planning application. Subsequent research has corroborated the power of the data collected with the care planning system by demonstrating its value in benchmarking and the identification of nursing best practices. Most disheartening is that nurses in the organizations referred to above anecdotally acknowledge that they complete care plan documentation in EHRs mainly to meet Joint Commission and other external standard requirements rather than to support quality and efficient patient care.

There were a number of failure points in the case described above but most link directly back to the fact that the parties involved based their decisions on insufficient information and faulty assumptions. When the model system was studied, it was common knowledge that implementing care plans and their documentation was problematic and no major EHR vendor had effectively addressed this problem.

Nurses wrongly assumed that technical barriers prevented the study tool from connecting to their EHRs and ceased to advocate for its implementation or continued use. The nurses also failed by not demanding that the chief health information system decision makers provide evidence to support the assertions about the future development and functionality of the EHRs. Instead the nurses assumed that the decision makers were operating with sufficient knowledge about workflow and care management systems; the nurses did not recognize that it was unrealistic to expect those who are not nurses to make high quality decisions about point-of-care work without ample input from the nurses who would be affected.

The chief health information system decision makers failed to recognize the complexity of the very costly decisions with which they were charged and the limitations of their own knowledge. The information technology leaders discounted the preferences of the nurses and made assurances that could not be fulfilled. Although engineering, computer, and information experts are needed to build EHRs, these experts are not clinicians and thus do not possess the clinical knowledge necessary to build or select high quality EHRs.

In conclusion, electronic health records are very complex systems and as such require the coordination of many different types of expertise to build, test, select, and implement point-of-care meaningful use. This case also provides an example of how poor outcomes can occur when stakeholders fail to take responsibility for those aspects of the EHR that are within their domains of skills and knowledge. The decision makers clearly operated outside their scope of knowledge by not seeking a better understanding of the vendor care planning systems and by discounting the vital input of the nurses. The nurses on the other hand failed by abdicating responsibility to decision makers without demanding that they provide convincing evidence of the espoused care planning capabilities of the vendor EHRs.

 Editor's Commentary

The author correctly notes that EHR initiatives are complex and require teams of individuals with diverse expertise. Technical, clinical, and project management leadership are all required for a successful EHR project. EHRs are first and foremost clinical initiatives, so clinical leadership must have a critical role in all decision making. However, other factors contribute to decisions about information technology strategies in a health system.

Some possible causative factors in this case:

- The executive management at the involved hospitals recognized the value of the care planning and documentation application, but was concerned about deploying a research system into a production healthcare services environment without a well-resourced support team and plan.

- The executive management was concerned about how issues found in the system would be resolved, or how the product would be further developed to meet evolving needs of nursing care planning and documentation.

- There were concerns about training and implementation tools to support a large-scale rollout of the application beyond the original four research sites.

- The research application had not been sufficiently tested against security threats.

- The creators of the application were not prepared to defend themselves against potential liability claims in case of adverse events involving the software or its performance.

- The development costs of the new system were estimated to be much more than those involved in implementing a vendor-based system.

If executive or information technology management decides not to deploy a system preferred or requested by clinician leaders, the decision must be carefully thought through and then communicated effectively to the clinician leaders and staff. Buy-in for decisions about which technologies not to implement can be as critical as buy-in for decisions about which are being implemented. Effective and open discussions about strategic health IT strategies are critical to maintaining the allegiance and commitment of all members of a hospital community. Since all health IT decisions involve trade-offs on some level, ignoring the open discussion and not reaching consensus about key strategies will create difficulties when implementing future systems. Without adoption of information systems, meaningful use of those systems cannot be achieved. Even specific trade-offs that affect quality of patient care may be supported by clinicians if these trade-offs contribute to a more effective, higher quality of care health system overall.

 Lessons Learned

- Integrate clinicians with adequate knowledge about point-of-care processes in the governance of EHR selections and implementations.
- Validate vendor's claims about functionality.
- Determine when integration of disparate solutions is preferable to a single integrated system.

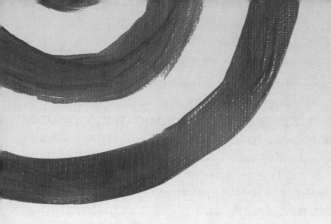

13

Lessons beyond Bar Coding: Lab Automation and Custom Development

Editor: Edward Wu

Key Words:	Project Categories:	Lessons Learned Categories:
bar code, internal development, interoperability, laboratory information system, pathology, patient safety, workflow	inpatient electronic health record (EHR), laboratory information systems	implementation approaches, project management, system configuration, system design, training, workflow

 Case Study

In a typical pathology laboratory, there are many so-called "assets" that need to be identified and tracked. These include requisitions with laboratory test orders as well as patient specimens and their derivatives, such as tissue blocks and glass slides. Deploying bar code solutions to track specimens has improved automation, efficiency, traceability, and patient safety. However, the use of bar code technology in the anatomic pathology laboratory is only a recent trend. This is largely due to a lack of available vendor solutions for use in the laboratory.

As a result of increasing asset volume and growing emphasis on patient safety, five years ago the anatomic pathology laboratory at a hospital embarked on implementing a bar code solution. As a result of this project, they were one of the first laboratories in the United States to transition from a manual, batch model operation to one that employed automated, real-time bar code tracking.

Prior to bar code implementation, tissue specimens were received in the laboratory with handwritten labels. Ideally specimens were accompanied by paper requisitions with patient details and physician instructions. Implementing bar coding at this stage was outside the purview of the laboratory. At the receiving area, laboratory employees manually entered cases or accessioned them into the laboratory information system (LIS), after which they were assigned a unique number. Introduction of bar coding at this step helped alleviate downstream specimen and paper mismatches, as well as the need for manual key entry of the case number and other details into the LIS.

Accessioned cases were passed on to prosectors who dissected the specimens into smaller tissue pieces to be placed within plastic cassettes. Previously, the case number and tissue key code were either handwritten or printed onto the cassettes. When prosectors transitioned to bar codes, the correct patient case immediately opened up in the LIS at their workstation. By printing bar codes directly on to the tissue cassettes (as seen in figure 13.1) only when needed, fewer mix-ups occurred.

At later stages of tissue processing, histotechnologists cut thin tissue sections for mounting on a glass slide. Bar coding these slides (as seen in figure 13.1) not only helped avoid mismatches, but helped drive protocols that standardized workflow (for example, laboratory personnel determined the

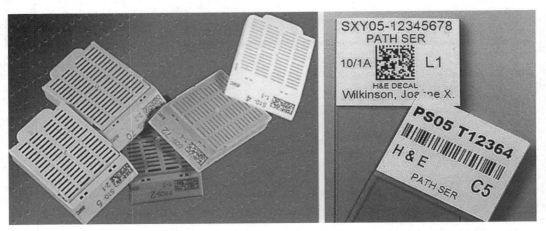

Figure 13.1. (Left) Plastic tissue cassettes with robust 2D bar codes embedded into the material. (Right) Examples of 1D (linear) and 2D (matrix code) laser-etched bar codes used to identify and track glass slides in the laboratory.

exact number of sections to be cut for particular biopsies). Because over one million slides are processed per year, mislabeling errors were a major concern. A labeling error could translate into a false positive cancer diagnosis, which would have been unacceptable.

Development of a practical and scalable bar coding solution for the laboratory was challenging and took over three years to accomplish. This was largely due to the limited ability of vendors to integrate bar coding solutions. The current LIS vendor was interested in participating, but did not have any of the necessary hardware (such as bar code scanners). Vendors for some of the instruments were also interested, but had not yet dealt with bar code technology. The vendor selected to supply bar coding hardware did not have software that was compatible with the current LIS. As there were no off-the-shelf solutions available, it was decided to utilize an internally developed bar code solution.

Despite adequate planning and sound IT project management, this venture was plagued with unexpected trials and tribulations. Much dialogue ensued around what data bar codes would contain, what they would look like, and where they would go. Prior to implementation of bar coding, case accession number and block designation were on the slide label. With the implementation of bar coding, laboratory personnel wanted to keep the same information on the labels and this had to be carefully balanced within the label and font-size constraints of the bar coded labels. Several trials were required to produce the optimal label with the correct font size and an acceptable human readability component alongside the bar code. The end result was a compromise that needed to be reached between employing a robust and a scalable bar code that was still readable to the human eye. In addition to the involvement by vendors, additional consultants with the necessary technical skills had to be brought together to help integrate the information from different systems into a single bar code. This was easier said than done, and resulted in a seemingly endless series of meetings and unsuccessful attempts to get the vendors to participate in an integrated single bar code. While the consultants' knowledge was helpful, the added layer of coordination added complexity that increased and compounded delays.

Overall, due to these delays and escalating costs, there was increased resistance from senior administration who wanted an explanation of ongoing expenditures to fix something they perceived was not broken. Additionally, histology laboratory staff were resistant to change and felt that bar coding was being implemented because of internal errors. They were also concerned that the new way of producing labels would require extra time and effort, which would introduce delays in their workflow.

After a pilot implementation involving one laboratory component, bar coding was rolled out to the entire laboratory in a stepwise fashion in three of the major medical centers. It soon became evident that the bar coding efforts increased efficiency and decreased labeling errors. For example, at one medical center the number of mislabeled slides fell from 12 per month to zero per month within six months of implementation. At another hospital three mislabeled slide events were encountered six months after implementation. This was attributed to a technologist using bar code labels in batches, instead of real time. Applying this batch of labels to the various assets led to mislabeling events.

However, the histotechnologists at a separate lab complained that their work was now taking much longer to complete, because they were being forced to work with only one case at a time, instead of batching their tasks. Staff training and education efforts were increased, leading to increased comfort with the change, expansion of bar coding efforts, and many other laboratories around the country following suit. Adoption of specimen tracking technology has not only proved useful for asset management and error reduction, but has also helped standardize workflow, supported lab automation, improved overall turnaround times, and driven our workflow processes in an efficient fashion.

 ## Author's Analysis

There is no true "plug and play" in the healthcare environment. To this day, a universal bar code with interoperability in the laboratory is still not available on the market. While the hospital was developing a customized solution for the laboratory, vendors were simultaneously developing products of their own, which caused unnecessary friction and delays to the project. To avoid such a situation, it is recommended that all parties clearly state their role, describe their current capabilities, and make sure there are no competing interests up front. The pilot project of bar coding one component of the laboratory was a very helpful step toward a successful implementation. The staff learned that it was not necessary to bar code every single asset in the laboratory to obtain a substantial improvement in both efficiency and patient safety. To the contrary, a phased implementation often renders more favorable results, in that the reduced scope of the overall project confers greater likelihood of initial success and user acceptance.

Because this project was so novel for the laboratory, it was difficult to plan ahead and be proactive regarding some project details. Project issues would emerge and need to be resolved quickly—hence the importance of paying attention to the details of a project in uncharted territory. Additionally, with complex and protracted projects, these details had the tendency to erode morale. Sometimes it proved more important to do things quickly rather than flawlessly.

Buy-in of all stakeholders is a key component to successful IT implementation. While informatics-related technologies may offer celebrated benefits, all parties should be aware of the operational burden they may place on overall workflow. Introducing bar coding into the laboratory was initially stressful for all workers. This was not surprising as implementing new IT or systems often means significant changes to workflow, working relationships, and other aspects of employees' daily routines. The success of an organizational change requires buy-in from all stakeholders. Therefore, it is important to make sure all staff feel empowered and understand that they are part of the solution.

Human noncompliance rather than technological issues may cause IT solutions to fail. Implementation of bar coding alone without user compliance can be problematic. In order to improve the quality of the service, it became necessary to change current operational processes. In this laboratory, that meant that some of the manual, batch-type tasks that histotechnologists performed had to be modified, even if it took them longer to complete only one task at a time.

 Editor's Commentary

Bar coding has proven to be an effective way to process goods or objects through a system. In the retail sector, it has been one of the most influential technological advances, offering great gains in efficiency. However, the use of bar coding in healthcare continues to mature, as this case illustrates. The author has described three key challenges to the adoption of bar coding: a lack of integration standards, the limitations of vendor support, and the need for substantial process change.

Because of the lack of integration standards, it was extremely difficult to find anything close to a "vendor-ready" solution. Had standards for bar code integration existed, vendors could more easily work with the author in the implementation. Instead, an internally developed strategy was required, posing a situation with inherent risks. For instance, the quality and upkeep of coding are typical challenges that arise in such a development environment. Internal development here led to a protracted project and complex issues that could not be foreseen.

Vendor cooperation was limited, and there may be multiple reasons why. Vendors, with their own schedules and motivations, may not have been aligned with the interests of the healthcare organization. As this case and many others have demonstrated, vendors like to stick to what they know best. Pushing into bar code technology would throw vendors into an area of uncertainty. Even if a vendor wished to cooperate, the high degree of customization would likely not make it economically feasible, at least initially, for continued cooperation on the project. Finally, vendors typically like to limit legal liability, and venturing into bar coding may have been too risky for them.

A third hurdle that the authors faced was the need for substantial process change. As with the implementation of any technology, ensuring adherence to proper processes is essential. It was identified that technicians should be processing samples one at a time using the new system. However, after bar code implementation, technicians reverted back to the batching of samples, which introduced error into the process. Specimens may have slipped into a batch unnoticed or may have gotten mixed up after scanning. Fortunately, the authors identified these challenges quickly and emphasized the importance of retraining on this essential process change. A key lesson here is that training, monitoring of processes, and retraining are all essential components to sustaining the momentum of technology implementations.

 Lessons Learned

- Internal development of software solutions is time-consuming and requires adequate development expertise.
- If there is not a vendor-ready solution vendors may not be aligned with end-user goals.
- Process change requires monitoring, training, and retraining.
- Phased approaches to bar code solutions can minimize impacts to workflow.

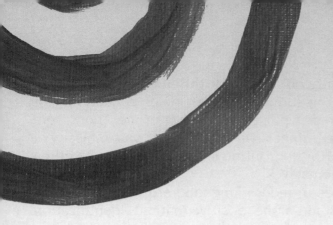

Sticker Shock: A Laboratory Information System

Editor: Edward Wu

Key Words:	**Project Categories:**	**Lessons Learned Categories:**
laboratory, stakeholder, custom development, scope	inpatient electronic health record (EHR), laboratory information systems	communication, leadership/governance, project management, system design, workflow

 Case Study

With the sponsorship of the chief quality officer, associate chief nurse, director of clinical pathology, and chief information officer (CIO), the executive management team at a major teaching hospital approved a project to build a closed-loop laboratory order management system. This teaching hospital has had a strong history of developing informatics solutions to improve patient safety and quality, and had been an early and successful adopter of computerized physician order entry (CPOE) and bar code medication administration (BCMA) technologies. However, more than 10 years into the adoption of CPOE, there was still no direct electronic communication between the fully deployed CPOE system and laboratory information system (LIS). Laboratory orders still required transcription to a paper laboratory requisition form by either the unit coordinator or the nurse. The rounding phlebotomist would then review this form prior to specimen collection. Not only were the many steps involved inefficient and error-prone, there were compliance concerns as physician trainees (who entered the vast majority of orders) routinely bypassed CPOE for nonroutine laboratory orders by filling out the paper requisition form themselves.

Encouraged by recent successes in redesigning laboratory CPOE screens and the implementation of a stand-alone positive patient identification (PPID) system (that is, scanning of patient wristbands resulting in bedside-generated specimen labels), a project team was assembled to develop an optimal electronic order communication system that would link the lab testing processes from order entry to result retrieval. The sponsors identified a physician, nurse, and a pathologist, each with significant experience with leadership and information technology projects, to colead the project. An experienced project manager was assigned full time to the project. Additionally, clinical systems analysts and application developers assisted with discovery, workflow analysis, and software design.

At the project kickoff meeting, a senior analyst presented the processes that could be addressed by an information technology solution, including duplicate laboratory order checking, assignment of specimen collection (to either nursing or phlebotomy), integration with PPID, merging of laboratory orders to minimize patient blood draws, workflow queue management for phlebotomy staff, and automatic request for specimen redraw if the first specimen is found to be unsatisfactory. A draft project charter listed nearly 15 project benefits and nearly 25 high-level business objectives. While the work ahead seemed daunting, the benefits of the project were evident to every member of the steering committee.

Early project discussions focused on coming to agreement on the scope and business objectives of the project, which took five months to finalize. The project team spent significant time understanding the current workflows across all stakeholders. With that in mind, the project team began to explore ways to deliver the project in phases with the hope that each phase would provide incremental benefit to the organization. Unfortunately, the project team was unable to address just a subset of the business requirements without negatively impacting the workflow of at least one key stakeholder group. Direction from the project sponsors at this point was to focus on all the business requirements to drive the technical design. The project team therefore focused its efforts on defining the future state workflows across all the major and minor stakeholders. With the help of a resident performance improvement team conversant in Lean and Six Sigma methodologies, the team organized two days of multistakeholder sessions, which resulted in high-level agreement for a combined future state workflow—more than 15 months after the project was kicked off.

The project information technology personnel, who had been following the workflow discussions and exploring technical approaches in the background, were then asked to define the architectural design and estimate the associated work effort. After more than 50 hours of deliberations involving multiple senior level IT personnel, it was determined that it would take a team of three analysts and four developers approximately four years to fully specify, develop, test, and implement the solution. The business owners were then asked again to explore ways to break up the deliverable into phases, but no agreement was reached out of concern that intermediate deliverables would cause significant workflow disruptions. The four-year timeline was brought to the project steering committee, which expressed concern regarding the significant time and resource commitments. Given the uncertainty about the future of the current clinical systems platform and the lack of ongoing support for a custom-developed system, the steering committee decided to put the project "on hold" 18 months after the project kickoff.

 Author's Analysis

Had the project sponsors recognized the level of complexity at the outset, they might have steered the project team differently. One early clue to the complexity was the high number of processes that the project set out to address through automation. Another red flag for complexity was the trio of key stakeholders (physician, nursing, and laboratory personnel) who needed to make decisions jointly regarding workflow. While the actions of any one group in large organizations are almost certain to have downstream effects, the amount of time and effort required to achieve consensus to change workflow and behavior likely goes up exponentially with the number of stakeholders involved. Lastly the high number of business objectives and benefits should have served as a warning signal of the project's complexity to the sponsors.

So what could have been done to manage a complex project such as this? A phased approach was a very reasonable strategy—the organization itself took this approach when it redesigned the laboratory order entry screen and deployed a stand-alone version of PPID before tackling the laboratory order communication project. By delivering partial solutions serially, projects can often become more "agile" by responding to changing business conditions and needs. This approach was however unsuccessful in the current project partly because the sponsors were not able to help the three main stakeholder groups identify a subset of business objectives the project team should focus on. An opportunity was also missed when the project team dismissed "lesser" solutions other hospitals had developed to link the laboratory orders between their CPOE and LIS systems. In retrospect, the project team could have achieved more if they had set more modest goals.

Executive leadership is often called upon to help projects move past their challenges. At times, it may need to set the expectation that compromises are needed to achieve organizational goals. At others, it may need to make unpopular decisions. When consensus cannot be reached across stakeholders, leadership may need to designate either itself or one of the stakeholders as the decision maker. Constraints to the project teams need to be articulated early on in the project and reinforced with key stakeholders, particularly when the scope of the solution threatens to become unmanageable. When the number of business objectives becomes overwhelming, leadership needs to prioritize them and jettison the less critical ones, or at least provide a framework for the project team so that the team has guidance in making difficult choices.

This case also serves to illustrate the risks associated with internal custom software development. While custom development is more likely to yield solutions that fit local culture and workflow, it tends to anchor staff in existing practices. In the desire to meet the needs of their constituents, custom development projects may struggle with scope, as the current project did. When the organization takes on this approach, it may need to invest in the necessary resources and organizational focus to support the product development cycle, such as the ability to try out small solutions and iterate on improvements over time before rollout of the product.

Finally, when a project can no longer meet its objectives given current business conditions, cancellation should not only be seen as a reasonable but also a desirable project outcome. When projects are cancelled, it is important for lessons learned to be captured and disseminated, and staff must be given the opportunity to apply their talents and skills towards other endeavors in the organization.

 ## Editor's Commentary

The author describes a project in which communication, scope complexity, and project management could have been enhanced. Due to limitations in these areas, project sponsors did not have a full picture of the project, which ultimately wasted the time and effort of many individuals.

Communication among project coleads, the steering committee, and IT leadership may have been inadequate for such a complex endeavor. A project this vast, with its broad goals and numerous stakeholders, needs frequent and open communication. The fact that project sponsors took 18 months to fully grasp resource requirements implies that communication could have been markedly improved. If key IT leaders were involved in early project discussions, this project would have been assessed in a more efficient and appropriate manner.

The author identifies scope complexity as a major red flag. Workflow analyses across physician, nursing, and laboratory areas were critical to understanding the scope and impact of this project. Unfortunately, it seemed that these analyses led to an increase in scope complexity. In many projects, scope complexity is mitigated utilizing project phases. The fact that a phased approach was unacceptable for the project sponsors ultimately led to its cancellation.

The project manager in this case may have managed project details well, but needed to be more up front about communicating scope complexity. Ideally, the project manager should have been in constant communication with project coleaders, so that escalation to project sponsors and IT leadership could have taken place much earlier.

In summary, this excellent case illustrates the need to communicate complexity to key stakeholders, and can serve as a lesson for any clinical systems project. While it did take 18 months to identify true project risks, the project sponsors are to be commended for putting this project "on hold." Even worse would have been to go forward with so much complexity and uncertainty regarding the future of the organization's clinical systems.

 Lessons Learned

- In any clinical systems project, involve key clinical and IT leaders.
- Understand and communicate project scope complexity, early and often.
- Establish project milestones with defined time periods and monitor for adherence.
- If possible, utilize a phased approach if a project scope is too large to implement at once.

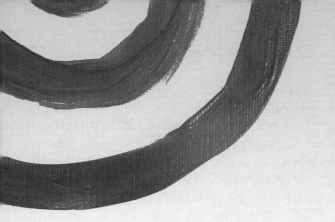

If It Ain't Broke, Don't Fix It: Replacing an HIS

Editor: Larry Ozeran

Key Words:	Project Categories:	Lessons Learned Categories:
best of breed, challenge assumptions, portal, open architecture, single-vendor solution, strategy, workflow	inpatient electronic health record (EHR)	leadership/governance, system design, workflow

 Case Study

Prompted by the inaugural staffing of its new chief information officer (CIO) position (after a two-year search), our large academic medical center reassessed the best-of-breed clinical information systems strategy it had pursued previously. We had implemented an open-architecture clinical data repository with an efficient portal for clinicians to review repository data, maintaining access to data in other systems. Under the new direction, we would actively pursue a single-vendor strategy as much as possible.

A request for proposal (RFP) was issued, and respondents were culled to a "short list" of major vendors offering large product suites. Each vendor gave an in-house demonstration, and each vendor's premier client site was visited. Participants in the demonstrations and visits (principally clinicians of all stripes and a range of administrators) provided feedback to an RFP evaluation committee, the majority of whom were administrators. The clinicians' strong consensus was that Vendor X's system (using a relatively closed architecture) had the least functional and least efficient clinician portal, nursing documentation system, and clinical data repository, whereas Vendor Y—supplier of the institution's existing systems in these areas—had the strongest products. However, because of the range of other products in the solution set it offered, as well as other administrative considerations (for example, larger company size), Vendor X was selected by the committee.

First, the institution's obsolete best-of-breed pharmacy system was replaced with Vendor X's pharmacy system. Next, development was undertaken simultaneously on Vendor X's nursing system, clinician portal, and clinical data repository (replacing Vendor Y's equivalent systems). Because it initially appeared that information entered into Vendor X's nursing system could be viewed only in Vendor X's portal, plans were made to deploy both systems in tandem on a ward-by-ward basis over a period of several weeks.

Concerns developed during the local development and configuration of Vendor X's nursing and portal systems, which seemed unimproved since the RFP demonstrations three years earlier. Casual testing of the impact of switching from Vendor Y's portal to Vendor X's portal demonstrated a significant loss of clinician efficiency. The time required to retrieve and understand a given body of results varied from approximately twofold to tenfold depending on the extent of the result set. Clinicians were concerned that without the luxury of seeing fewer patients, their existing limited time for data review might potentially result in diagnostic and therapeutic delays and errors.

Nevertheless, to promote the institutional benefits of a single-vendor strategy, we activated the new repository and began to implement the nursing and portal systems. Nurses indicated that their new system was weaker than Vendor Y's system but was tolerable. Physician portal users (including residents, physician extenders, and medical students) expressed substantial dislike for their new portal, but it was hoped that this assessment was merely an adjustment reaction. Implementation proceeded throughout the wards, with clinicians making workflow adjustments as necessary (for example, rounding without information on current vital signs because data collection was either too time-consuming or in fact impossible). However, on the first attempt to go live in one of the intensive care units, the new portal's deficiencies led to a serious reduction in patient care quality. The intensivists' understanding of their patients' conditions deteriorated so precipitously that go-live was halted after four days, workflow was reverted to prior procedures, and further analysis was undertaken to determine if the product's deficiencies could be satisfactorily addressed.

Analysis showed that the new portal's deficiencies could not be rectified using the current version of the product. Discussions with the vendor indicated that sufficient improvements would not be available for at least a few years.

The new portal was deemed an institutional failure.

Alternative approaches were quickly identified and evaluated. One option was to adopt the latest version of Vendor Y's product, a substantial enhancement over our older version; we had deferred numerous upgrades because of uncertainty about our strategy. After 15 years successfully interfacing numerous ancillary systems to Vendor Y's open architecture portal, we found that Vendor X's ancillary systems (for example, nursing and medication administration) could be interfaced to Vendor Y's portal. The clinical community again concluded Vendor Y's portal was the preferred product. Leadership nimbly switched gears and struck a deal with Vendor Y to rapidly implement not only its upgraded portal but also some newer modules, including an open architecture clinical data mining package that will serve not only our institution but also a developing statewide consortium of academic medical centers. Our decision to retain an open architecture repository was soon serendipitously reinforced by the emergence of an independently developed plan for a health information exchange in which clinical systems from our institution and several regional competitors will be linked to improve patient care.

 ## Author's Analysis

Many lessons have been learned or reinforced during this odyssey. Our "top five" are as follows:

First, "don't fix what ain't broke." Vendor Y's systems had long worked well. Their architecture was well suited to an academic environment in need of best-of-breed ancillary systems and was highly efficient for review of the voluminous data pool created by testing performed on complex tertiary patients. Vendor X's portal was determined early on to be significantly inferior to Vendor Y's portal for our needs. In retrospect, a more careful consideration of the possibility of continuing to use Vendor Y's portal may have helped.

Second, busy clinicians highly value their time and thus prize tools that improve their efficiency. Clinicians' needs are served well by carefully assessing in advance the efficiency of new tools proposed for their use. Tools for clinicians that do not improve efficiency should be examined critically prior to adoption; tools that significantly worsen efficiency require remarkable benefits elsewhere in the organization to justify adoption.

Third, user opinion ("the will of the people") is discounted at one's peril. Clinicians who previewed Vendor X's suite during the RFP demonstrations were unanimously opposed to their portal, an opinion discounted by the administrator-heavy RFP evaluation committee. In retrospect, it was not surprising (and thus avoidable) that Vendor X's portal was poorly received during initial implementation and ultimately deemed a failure.

Fourth, understanding expectations prior to deployment of a new system can help avoid disappointments and failures. Vendor X was perplexed by our dislike for its portal. They claimed that all of their other customers had received it well, but admitted those customers had never had a portal before, possibly facilitating their perception of Vendor X's portal as an improvement. Also, Vendor X never analyzed Vendor Y's portal and our clinicians' use of it, thus failing to discover in advance that the replacement would be a net down-grade. As soon as it became apparent that improvement was not forthcoming, disappointment and failure became highly likely.

Fifth, flexibility is crucial. As portal implementation was ultimately unsuc-cessful, we discovered centers similar to ours that had learned to use Vendor X's nonportal products with their own portals. Rather than persist with an inef-fective portal, our leadership quickly leveraged this discovery and switched to a more successful path.

We hope other healthcare institutions—and HIT vendors—will learn from our experience and avoid similar errors in the future.

 ## Editor's Commentary

Where to begin? So many things went wrong and yet the overlying answer should be to challenge your assumptions. The CIO assumed that a single-vendor solution would be better than a multivendor approach. When things weren't going well, that would have been a good time to reassess. Hospital administration assumed that clinicians would overcome their dislike of the system and be compliant with whatever the institution bought. There was an assumption that the portal would improve in the three years from demonstration of the product to its implementation. Clinicians assumed they could not spend more time reviewing the data but would have a new workflow option (for example, chart printout). In addition to other assumptions, the information technology department assumed that the new vendor's modules could be implemented in phases, but the advantage of a single vendor became problematic, and some modules were dependent on the existence of others.

The authors should be applauded for sharing this story because there is anecdotal evidence suggesting that this scenario occurs frequently but few are willing to talk about it. The most difficult aspect of challenging your assumptions is realizing that you are making an assumption. This is where it can be helpful to identify knowledgeable, reliable, honest people within your organization to ask periodically if what you are doing still makes sense. Make those queries part of your process by making them an appointment on your project timeline and plan. Ongoing bidirectional communication is a critical element of success. Keep open the lines of communication with all stakeholders. When there is significant disagreement among stakeholders, as happened in this case study, consider bringing in an experienced consultant to provide an independent point of view. However, when the stakeholders who are expected to use the system are overruled by those who manage the system, beware.

 Lessons Learned

- "Don't fix what ain't broke."
- Remember that clinicians prize tools that improve efficiency.
- Do not discount clinician input.
- Understand expectations prior to technology deployment.
- Always keep open lines of communication.
- Be flexible.

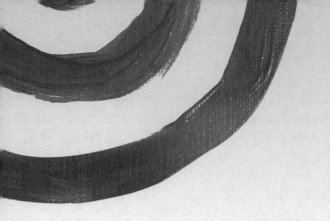

CHAPTER 16

A Single Point of Failure: Protecting the Data Center

Editor: Bonnie Kaplan

Key Words:	Project Categories:	Lessons Learned Categories:
business continuity, computerized provider order entry (CPOE), data center, downtime, environmental threats	infrastructure and technology	project management, technology problems

 Case Study

Tertiary medical institutions typically centralize most of their mission-critical clinical data in a central data center, which is a single physical location that is closely monitored for temperature, humidity, and the presence of smoke, fire, or flooding to prevent catastrophic failures.

When sensors detect specified deviations from environmental norms, a number of protocols are initiated with the goal of minimizing data loss. These protocols include orderly shutdown of the data servers, subsequent discontinuation of electric power, proactive mitigation of environmental threats (such as the release of fire suppressants), and computer notification (via pager) to specified on-call data center personnel.

The following two examples describe incidents involving the automatic shutdown of the central data center at an urban tertiary care academic institution when sensors detected aberrant conditions. The data center contains production databases for an institution-wide intranet server and systems for institution-wide electronic medical records, CPOE, pharmacy dispensing, admission-discharge-transfer (ADT), and intensive care unit (ICU) clinical documentation.

Example 1

In 2005, a failure of the data center fire alarm system occurred; a piece of plastic within the housing of the wall-mounted fire alarm broke. (The manufacturing cost of the failing piece was less than $1.) This resulted in the triggering of the fire alarm with a subsequent programmed, orderly shutdown of all servers, discontinuation of electric power, and release of the fire suppressant agent Halon into the data center.

For several hours, all data center services were unavailable, and providers had to switch to paper-based ordering and charting until the emergent problem was handled. Once the source of the alarm was identified and the Halon was cleared, the clinical data systems were restarted without data loss and with resumption of normal function.

Example 2

Two years later, a weekend water outage in the building housing the data center was scheduled by the maintenance staff, but was not properly communicated to the engineering staff. Despite a clearly posted policy to the contrary, maintenance staff disabled a primary water pump supplying water to the building.

The water outage interrupted the chilled water supply to the data center air handlers and resulted in a malfunction, which in turn shut down the air conditioning in the building. This resulted in a rise in environmental temperature that was detected by sensors, resulting in a programmed shutdown of the clinical servers, followed by discontinuation of electric power to the data center. Because the smoke alarm was not triggered, the fire suppression agent was not released.

Data center personnel were notified immediately of the shutdown, but its cause (air conditioning failure due to the water outage) was not immediately apparent. After several hours, water services were restored, the air conditioning was restarted, and the temperature in the data center was normalized. The clinical data systems servers were restarted without data loss.

The water outage (and the resulting cascade of air conditioning failure and data center outage) forced the clinical staff to revert to paper ordering and charting. The incident resulted in no apparent patient harm, but lack of complete and accurate data was found to be a major user concern when the incident was reviewed by an institutional committee.

 ## Author's Analysis

Closed loop systems (as described in the data center environmental protection system in the previous examples) automate system responses (system shutdown, threat mitigation, and staff alert) to specified rules from defined input (abnormal environmental variables). In high-risk industries such as aeronautics and nuclear power, they are used to aid human operators (who in turn override inappropriate machine responses). In clinical care, they have been used to control experimental insulin pumps, pacemakers, and anesthesia machines, but sparingly, because of inherent risks.

"Who monitors the monitors?" is an apt question regarding the design of closed loop systems in enterprise health information systems. The increasing reliance on clinical information technology systems (since this scenario from 2007, CPOE use within the health system has increased to 80 percent of all physician orders) makes unanticipated outages (even short ones), as described in the foregoing examples, highly disruptive to continuity of care and may jeopardize patient care with errors of omission or commission and preventable delays.

Clinical data centers must ensure information (its confidentiality, integrity, and availability) with minimal unplanned downtime. With robust designs, unplanned outages are usually minimal, and closed loop environmental monitors, as described in the examples, usually work well, thus not warranting human surveillance. However, current designs are limited to a few independent data measurements and cannot distinguish between a true threat and an internal monitoring failure. The data center monitoring system was originally implemented with the assumption that shutting down the servers in an emergency is preferable (even in error) to data loss from continued operation resulting in permanent damage. With increasing institutional reliance, the error of commission was becoming increasingly problematic and disruptive.

What can be learned from these outages?

Data centers are "single points of failure" that are protected by monitoring systems that shut down according to a predefined set of rules that have thresholds.

The acceptability of these thresholds may change over time because of changes in institutional dependence on the data center, which may require reassessment of failure modes and their acceptability.

Planning of protection responses may require consideration of unanticipated "normal" events external to the data center with override rules, workaround protocols, and timely and appropriate human interventions.

In the case of the described institution, a remote redundant secondary data center was built. Clinical systems are now configured to switch to the secondary data center automatically in a "near real-time" fashion in the event of an outage in the primary center.

Hospital administrators, IT staff, and vendors must be aware of how defense systems for data centers function and how they fail. They also should evolve these systems from experience. The design of redundant systems (backup environmental systems and power sources, alternative short-term data storage), "smart" closed loop systems that infer the likelihood of true threats based on multiple inputs, and critical defense protocols is key in maintaining system availability.

 Editor's Commentary

Both of the examples describe unanticipated ways that system failure occurs. Each time, sensors detected abnormalities that led to automatic shutdown of a data center. In the first example, an inexpensive plastic piece in the fire alarm housing broke. This triggered a fire alarm, a shutdown, and firefighting actions, even though there was no fire. In the second example, workers disabled a water pump and did not notify system engineers, despite clear policy to the contrary. The disabled pump caused an air conditioning failure, which then caused the system to shut down as the temperature rose past the cutoff point. In each example, staff reverted to manual medical record keeping with no apparent patient harm. However, staff were concerned about lack of complete and accurate data after the second incident. Because increasing system use would make system outages even more disruptive, a remote redundant secondary data center was established so that system functions would be switched there if an outage occurred at the primary center.

As the author points out, contingency planning and manual procedures are vital. The examples indicate how important it was to have staff able to switch to manual procedures when automated ones failed. Moreover, a wise decision was made when a secondary data center was established so that crucial system functions could be continued smoothly if the primary center fails. Even though problems could again occur at either the primary or secondary center, the likelihood of them occurring simultaneously at both centers is small.

Neverthless, as the examples amply show, all sorts of unanticipated things may happen. The examples also show that failures can occur for many inter-related reasons. As the author rightly says, it is not possible to respond correctly to all situations in systems by monitoring according to predefined rules. Thresholds need to be reevaluated periodically.

I think other potential safeguards also are suggested by these examples. Would it not be better to try reducing such alarms? In the first example, a plastic part broke, and that triggered the fire alarm, causing a several-hour shutdown. It was difficult to identify the cause of the problem. Perhaps routine parts inspections or replacements would have prevented the problem. Perhaps better awareness of vulnerabilities of this sort would have been helpful. Perhaps redundancy, such as noticing the lack of smoke or heat detection, would have helped.

The second example points even more strongly to a variety of interlocking causes and multiple failure points, leading to multiple possibilities for preventive measures. Policy violations meant that staff was not notified of the water outage, and that a crucial pump was disabled. Either workers were ignorant of the policy or disregarded it. Remedial action is needed, based on the reason for the policy violations. Workers could be better trained and the policy rationale better explained, or maybe the policy itself needs revision. The policy could be posted more clearly. A sign-off could be instituted when crucial functions are to be interrupted. If various utilities (water, electricity) are interrupted routinely, an alert system might be put in place to warn data center staff.

These are some possible ideas. Others might well make more sense. Without knowing the institution, those involved, and reasons for failure beyond those built into the automatic system, it is hard to make sound recommendations. Instead, the suggestions are meant to illustrate an important point when analyzing problematic situations. There are different ways to analyze causes of failure so as to remediate them. The focus can be on the system itself. Maybe hardware or software is to blame. In these examples, there clearly were system failures caused by automatic built-in responses. Reevaluating thresholds is one way to address this issue, as is having a secondary backup center. Alternatively, the focus can be on personnel. When policies are violated, new procedures and training can be instituted. In these examples, when the systems went down, patient care functions continued with limited loss of patient data or threats to patient safety because staff was well prepared and acted appropriately. Finally, the focus can be on how everything—system, personnel, and procedures—works together in inter-related ways, something these examples illustrate. Broadening "system" to include personnel and procedures as well as hardware and software could provide a wider perspective on how to better design safeguards. All three of these perspectives can help address failures.

The title of this chapter shortchanges the richness of these examples. Rather, the stories indicate multiple failure points and ways to address them.

 Lessons Learned

- Downtime management requires complex planning.
- System redundancy is required across all components of HIT.
- Automated alarms and processes must be appropriate to a specific environment.
- System interdependencies cannot be overestimated.
- Policies and procedures must include enforcement and training or retraining.
- Communication is crucial.

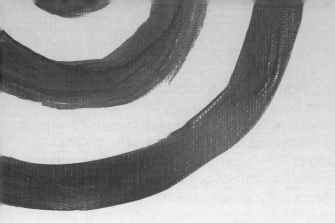

Vendor and Customer: Single Sign-On

Editor: Justin Graham

Key Words:	Project Categories:	Lessons Learned Categories:
context management, project management, single sign-on, software development, testing, workflow	inpatient electronic health record (EHR), infrastructure and technology	communication, implementation approaches, leadership/ governance, project management

 Case Study

A nationally prominent academic health system awarded a contract for single sign-on (SSO) and context management (CM). The health system was implementing new electronic health record (EHR) features including computerized provider order entry (CPOE) and the chief information officer (CIO) wanted to improve clinician workflow with SSO and CM first. The health system had conducted an extensive selection process that included an open request for proposals, vendor technology demonstrations, and reference calls to existing health systems using the technologies desired. The selection process revealed that no single vendor could provide a complete solution to the functional requirements desired by the health system, so the final contract required additional software development of the products to be implemented. A contract was signed and the project began.

After the project kickoff, the health system and technology vendor teams reviewed project plans and set up testing and development systems. Quickly, certain conflicts emerged in the project. The health system's CIO, a clinician, delegated the project to a junior, nonclinical, information technology (IT) manager and directed the vendor team to work with the designee and the IT team. The CIO was confident in the ability of the vendor and the IT teams to develop the right solution; the vendor team did not share the same confidence. The IT manager had a background in security technology but little experience in healthcare IT and had favored a different solution during the selection process. The project team did not include clinicians from the health system as the IT manager wanted to complete the SSO and CM configuration under management of the IT department and then present a finished solution to clinicians for implementation. Despite repeated requests from the vendor, the IT manager would not allow the vendor's development or implementation teams to engage health system clinicians during implementation. Because of this, the vendor team repeatedly advised leaders within the health system that the IT manager might not be qualified to make decisions that affected clinician workflows in clinical applications. The vendor team and the health system IT team disagreed about how to implement different functions of the SSO and CM technologies and which approaches would be preferable or even acceptable to clinicians, such as the speed-performance requirements for the SSO and CM software.

It was at this point that problems started to occur. The health system requested a formal testing plan that required a model configuration to be installed in the health system's testing infrastructure. The vendor provided the software, but without the full functionality previously communicated to the health system; the vendor continued development of the anticipated functionality and planned to make available a new software release with all the necessary functionality prior to the health system's go-live date for SSO and CM. Additionally, the health system's IT team was not able to configure its IT test environment according to the vendor's recommendations for optimal software performance. In the test system as configured, the SSO and CM software did not perform as the IT manager wanted, although the vendor team was pleased with the newly developed functionality. Throughout testing, the vendor continued the development process for the new software release, modifying the software iteratively as problems were encountered. The go-live date neared, preventing a full test scenario from being performed on a single set of code. Each step in testing was applied only to the most recent software installed at the time of the test. When code changes were made, there was no time to perform regression testing.

The vendor team maintained a project plan and tracked open issues that needed to be addressed; the project manager maintained a separate list of open issues to be addressed. Most but not all issues appeared on both lists. After continued conflicts between the vendor team and the health system's IT team about software performance and functionality, the SSO and CM software implementation was stopped. The vendor's executive team and the health system's CIO agreed the project would not go live.

 ## Author's Analysis

This biggest surprise of this project was that it proceeded as far as it did. Following the selection process, the health system should have recognized the challenges the SSO and CM project encompassed, especially because no commercially available product met the functional requirements. A reassessment of functional requirements, the desired timeline, or the dedicated project team might have mitigated sufficient risks and allowed a successful outcome. Instead, the health system forged ahead to implement "not-yet-available" software within a predefined timeframe. The health system partnered in the challenge of developing new software without recognizing it was not prepared to do so. The approach made the health system's larger HIT projects (including CPOE) dependent on a project that was itself precariously dependent on a vendor's ability to develop and deliver new software, the health system's ability to implement novel software, and the project supervision of a mid-level manager without appropriate healthcare workflow expertise. And, despite the admirable intent to perform adequate testing prior to implementation, the testing scenario protocols were flawed and failed to take into account the vendor's extensive ongoing software development.

The vendor, in turn, took a serious risk with a project that was likely to fail at a nationally prominent academic health system. The vendor recognized from the beginning some of the challenges resulting from the health system's approach, but did not recognize the likelihood of failure involved in developing and testing new software within the committed project timeline. The vendor was more focused on the potential benefits of successfully developing and implementing software at a prestigious health system, rather than the reality that these benefits were unlikely to be achieved with resultant negative backlash. The vendor should have said no to the unrealistic requests of the client rather than commit to deliver and then fail to do so.

Open collaborative communication to identify problems and resolve them was the missing safety net for this high risk HIT project; the conflicts between the health system IT team and the vendor team should have been sufficient flags to both groups that the project could not succeed. Perhaps the only successful outcome of this project was that both parties ultimately agreed that the project was going to fail, and the implementation was stopped before it was rolled out and further resources (or even patient lives) were lost. Sometimes stopping a project is the best next step.

Editor's Commentary

Custom software development is a high-risk endeavor for healthcare providers. Hospitals and health systems have business goals that revolve around optimizing patient care and meeting regulatory standards, goals that are often incompatible with the iterative cycles of requirements analysis, development, testing, and documentation that good software requires. The health system described in the case doubled down on this long shot by putting the SSO and CM project in the critical path for a major EHR rollout. Fortunately, they were wise enough to recognize their overreach and pull the plug on the software before it dragged their entire EHR project (and, likely, the health system's strategic plan) down with it.

Even if the software development had gone without a hitch, the chances of project success remained slim. In all likelihood, the health system would have soon learned that an IT project intended to radically alter clinical workflow would be doomed to failure if clinicians were not involved early in the process, if only to support change management efforts.

Lessons Learned

- Sometimes the best next step in a project is to stop.
- When customers ask for what a vendor cannot deliver, or cannot deliver without unacceptable risk, vendors should not be afraid to tell their clients "no."
- Involve clinicians early and often in projects that will affect their workflow.
- Extensive testing is essential to an HIT initiative's success.
- Vendor-customer development partnerships require effective leadership for both mutual respect and frequent open communication.

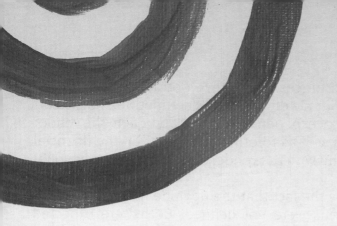

CHAPTER 18

Ready for the Upgrade: Upgrading a Hospital EHR for Meaningful Use

Editor: Edward Wu

Key Words:	Project Categories:	Lessons Learned Categories:
upgrade, cost overrun, vendor challenges, mock go-live, Meaningful Use upgrade	inpatient electronic health record (EHR), infrastructure and technology	communication, contracts, leadership/governance, project management

 Case Study

Hospital A had been on version X.X of the hospital's main EHR (electronic health record). Because of Meaningful Use (MU) requirements, they needed to implement a newer, MU-certified version of the software. However the vendor had not yet made that version available. The process was further complicated by the fact that they were two versions behind the certified version. The longstanding policy was to delay software upgrades or installations until other institutions had gone through a similar implementation. However, because of time constraints, and because they had uneventfully completed full upgrades and several incremental upgrades over the last several years, they decided to proceed.

Two options were then considered. The first would be to perform two separate and consecutive upgrades to the MU-certified version of the EHR, requiring twice the time and resources. The other option was to use an untested approach: perform an upgrade directly to the certified version as part of a single effort. Despite the lack of experience with this approach, the vendor recommended it to hospital A as well as to other clients. Given the financial and time pressures to meet MU and with the vendor's assurances, the hospital elected to pursue this option.

The choice was complicated by the fact that the upgrade had not yet been developed, and the contract terms were not defined. Both were expected within "a few weeks" of selecting our upgrade strategy. The longer the hospital waited for the vendor to be ready, the more they needed the efficiencies of the double upgrade. They contemplated reverting to the two-stage approach, but soon learned from other sites that this approach also had significant challenges. They eventually waited several months for contract negotiations to be completed and for the offering to be made available. There was further delay because the vendor resources were stretched very thin and could not be assigned to the hospital for several months after the execution of the contract.

Eventually the vendor and the hospital project team codeveloped the project charter and scope, as well as a work plan with milestones and dates. Three mock go-lives were planned in preparation for go-live: one in the Development domain, one in the Train domain, and the third in the Test domain.

First up was the mock go-live for Development (Mock 1). Unfortunately, the delivery of the development environment was delayed several weeks due to issues with vendor resources, deployment methods, and various software bugs. The delays in the validation, configuration, and testing of the Development environment infringed on the Train environment (Mock 2). The experience with Mock 2 was no different. Delivery of the environment was later than planned. Issues identified during Mock 1 recurred and new ones surfaced. The sense was that the upgrade process was unpredictable. Test (Mock 3) was also delayed significantly for similar reasons.

Because of the concerns, additional mock go-lives were planned. The hospital and vendor also decided that they would not pursue a production go-live until seven days of system stability (without any changes required) and a successful stress test was achieved.

Eventually five mock go-lives were required before the system was stable and worthy of placing in front of end-users for stress testing. Unfortunately, the stress testing also revealed bugs and slowness that were not seen with previous unit and integrated testing. Additional workarounds were employed, more fixes were loaded, and the stress tests were then repeated. However system slowness in several key areas prevented the scheduling of a Production go-live.

Throughout this upgrade process, the hospital had good communication with the vendor. Individuals from vendor leadership were engaged and on site during this entire process. Despite vendor involvement, hospital executive leadership decided to halt work on the upgrade. Consequently, the CEOs of the vendor and the hospital met to clarify the working relationship and address the upgrade problems at hand.

Taking a step back and addressing upgrade issues with the vendor was helpful. Over the next two months, fix after fix was successfully loaded. The vendor engaged development partners with expertise in the server and network platforms to improve critical login issues. Weeks of thorough investigation of the EHR resolved remaining functional issues with allergy documentation; and resequencing table entries solved another significant patient safety issue.

At last seven days of complete stability without the need for any system changes was achieved. The delays and "retrenching" ultimately cost the hospital several hundred thousand dollars plus the opportunity costs of not being able to focus on other important initiatives. So, with cost overruns and delayed timelines, the hospital finally went live with the upgrade—which was completely uneventful. Any glitches that occurred were invisible to the end-user and rapidly resolved by the vendor-client team.

Both the hospital and vendor put in an extraordinary numbers of hours to achieve this near flawless go-live. Despite the go-live success, the hospital did suffer in other areas due to this upgrade. Some system maintenance and enhancements were delayed, and regulatory updates were postponed.

In the end, we realized were it not for our extra effort, expense, and time, the end result would have been very different.

 Author's Analysis

In healthcare IT, our misses may be as important as our successes. The project management literature is littered with mantras like "if it's worth doing at all, then it is worth doing right the first time." But how much attention is given to the effort required to put a perfect process into production on the first attempt? When patient safety is at stake, not only is it worth doing right the first time, it is imperative.

Although eventually the go-live was nearly flawless, the events that led up to it was like a series of sports events—complete with trick plays, errors, and injuries. In fact, the hospital incurred immense cost overruns and had to delay other important projects in patient safety and regulatory initiatives. The hospital was successful only because of its own persistence and the vendor's shared commitment to the project.

Implementations are a complex undertaking for both customers and vendors. External regulatory pressures further complicate the picture for both customers and vendors, causing additional challenges. Internal pressures—in the form of capital improvements, patient safety initiatives, and personnel changes—can make an implementation extremely challenging.

In this case, we learned that multiple failures prior to go-live can provide important information that can lead to a flawless go-live. Key to this is that vendors and customers form a partnership to work though inevitable difficulties.

 ## Editor's Commentary

This case illustrates two major implementation missteps—not pushing a vendor to adhere to contract terms and fully trusting a vendor on a complicated upgrade. Vendor resources were not delivered as promised, and it became apparent that the vendor had very little expertise with the upgrade at hand. With a "double upgrade," the degree of difficulty goes up exponentially, and generally, most vendors have limited field experience in these situations. Ultimately, the hospital regained footing after these faults were escalated to hospital leadership.

To limit risks like this during an upgrade, three main components need to be addressed: vendor communication, key stakeholder communication, and appropriate project management.

In this case, vendor communication seemed to be going well, but the project was stalled until key hospital and vendor leadership convened. While not the norm, this is sometimes required to address risks at a senior leadership level. In fact, this may be the first time vendors learn what has been escalated to hospital executives. As readers we do not know exactly what occurred in this meeting, but it is likely that a great deal of risk mitigation and action plans were developed. Hospital leaders likely pushed vendors for hard deadlines (something that should have happened at the outset) and may have asked for additional vendor resources to complete the upgrades.

Communication to project sponsors and stakeholders should also take place to manage expectations. All but the most minor of upgrades should be communicated to key stakeholders. Not only do clinicians and administrators need to know the benefits of an upgrade, but they also need to be aware of downtime ramifications and potential changes to workflow. Keeping all leaders and end-users informed can manage expectations, mitigate potential downstream risks, and develop champions for the process. Additionally, involving key stakeholders early and often during an upgrade can uncover specific workflow issues that would not otherwise be addressed.

Most important to a software upgrade is appropriate project management. A software upgrade should be considered a project in and of itself. Scope, time, and resources need to be integrated into the decision to upgrade.

It can be extremely tempting to just run a patch with only minimal testing, communication, or resources—but that usually is a recipe for disaster. Thorough implementation, testing, and validation are necessary for the go-live of any major upgrade, much less a double upgrade performed in one step.

In this case, communication and project management were strong, but the project required escalation to hospital leadership to ensure success. Strengths of this implementation included the dedication to a "perfect go-live" with multiple mock go-lives and constant vendor communication, despite initial setbacks. Despite their success, it is likely that a "double upgrade" will be handled with even greater caution in the future.

 Lessons Learned

- Communication between vendor and hospital is necessary for successful upgrade implementation.
- Upgrades rarely go without a hitch, so good planning and ample communication can mitigate risks.
- Escalation to hospital and vendor leadership may be necessary if the project is not going well.
- If timelines are critical, contracts should include date milestones.

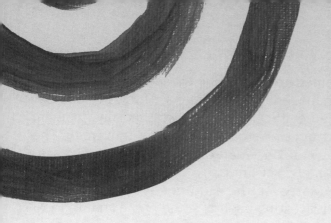

Effective Leadership Includes the Right People: Informatics Expertise

Editor: Gail Keenan

Key Words:	Project Categories:	Lessons Learned Categories:
change, electronic health record (EHR), informatics specialist, information technology (IT) decisions, organizational culture	inpatient electronic health record (EHR)	data model, leadership/ governance, system configuration

 Case Study

A long-standing medical college and hospital with a proud history of innovation, which nearly went bankrupt, was acquired and saved by a university and a national for-profit hospital chain company. The university acquiring the medical college lacked healthcare experience. The acquired hospital had been nonprofit in its century of existence, and the takeover by a for-profit chain was somewhat of a shock to its faculty and staff. The ultimate solution, however, was better than other alternatives discussed before the takeover—including turning the facility into condominiums.

Merging the cultures of the medical college and university was proving a challenge. A culture of mistrust and anxiety about cross-college collaborations with the acquiring university seemed to prevail at the medical college. It certainly did not help when a managerial and financial "firewall" was set up between the university and the healthcare campus, so that any financial trouble in the healthcare units would not cross over to the university. The acquired managed-care-owned hospital, once part of a proud and unified academic medical center, was now largely "off limits" to management of either the medical college or university. Moreover, the acquiring for-profit hospital chain owner was losing money and divesting itself of some of the chain's local hospitals.

A medical informatics specialist with significant experience in design and implementation of clinical IT in nearby large medical centers was hired by the main university, but with a primary appointment in a computer and information-related college and not the medical college. The informaticist was to develop an educational program in medical informatics to help set up cross-college collaborations in informatics research, and assist in other areas as needed.

The College of Medicine did not leverage the informaticist in the implementation of an electronic health record (EHR) for its for-profit faculty practice plan. The informaticist offered her services and the medical college's and faculty practice plan's dean, chief information officer (CIO), chief operations officer (COO), and other top executives were well aware of her background. Because of existing sociocultural issues that divided the acquired medical campus and the acquiring university (mostly in the domain of distrust—and perhaps disdain), the informaticist's services or advice were not utilized.

Here is a summarized report from an HIT blog:

> A posted record of lawsuit was filed against the EHR vendor by the University's College of Medicine's for-profit practice group, claiming that the EHR "does not function per the specifications provided." The lawsuit accused the vendor of breach of contract, fraud, and other contractual shortcomings. Over $1 million was paid for the system, and problems with claims billing cost the practice group twice that amount. The university filed an injunction requiring the EHR vendor to provide a system that performs evaluation and management (E/M or billing) coding or pay professional coders to do the job. One example they cited: no Review of Systems template existed for the E/M coder that handles allergy/immunologic or hematologic/lymphatic organ systems. They provided confirmation from the EHR vendor that certain aspects of the EHR did not function properly.

The informaticist had direct and relevant experience in EHR implementation and would have recommended extensive testing of the financial components before go-live. She had observed similar happenings at a different university, where a different faculty practice plan and vendor's defective products collided and resulted in a US Department of Justice investigation, a large fine, admission by the university that it lacked the appropriate IT management depth, and complete abandonment of a multimillion-dollar IT investment because of resultant defective billing practices.

 ## Author's Analysis

Informatics specialists should be aware of the challenges of integrating cultures of healthcare systems and nonhealthcare components of universities. Informatics experts should be aware that their expertise may be regarded as unneeded or perhaps frightening to officials in charge of EHR implementation, who often lack medical backgrounds and are being asked to do much more than they are really capable of doing. Informaticists should educate hospital and university officials that not knowing what you don't know about complex EHR issues, and placing too much trust in vendor promises, can lead to system failure—or worse.

 ## Editor's Commentary

The merging of very different cultures under a single umbrella is problematic, especially during the period immediately following a takeover. Moreover, if no plan or actions are taken to unify the diverse entities into a productive whole, the entities are likely to remain at odds indefinitely. This translates into employees working at cross purposes or not being utilized when appropriate, resulting in increasing associated costs. This seems to have been the situation described in the case study. It is unfortunate that the medical informatics specialist, given her background, was not tapped for her expertise in EHRs even though she offered assistance. In organizations with effective cultures, individuals recognize their strengths and weaknesses and do what it takes to find and utilize the best expertise to solve group problems. This did not happen in the organization described in the case study.

There are a number of possible perspectives that one might consider to achieve a better outcome in a similar situation; two will be discussed here. The first is to avoid working for organizations that have ineffective cultures. These actually can be spotted during the interview phase. It is recommended that one talk with as many potential colleagues in an organization to assess a match with the values and ways business is conducted and problems are solved. Colleagues at higher and lower levels as well as in departments with which one might expect to collaborate should be interviewed. If the fit seems poor, you are likely to be continually frustrated unless you hold a top position of influence within your area of expertise (or have the support of the person who does).

A second perspective would be to take the job but with a solid proactive approach about how you will work effectively within the organization to improve the culture. For example, as a condition for employment, you could stipulate in your contract that you would be given the option to serve as a member on all committees that focus on the EHR within the health-related colleges and affiliated hospitals. Also, you could begin to nurture relationships with colleagues of like mind who eventually could work together to move IT actions and policy in the desired direction.

There is one other consideration. Sometimes those responsible for making HIT decisions but unqualified to make those decisions are insecure in their positions, leading to their distrust of local experts. These leaders have no way of knowing whether the local expert is acting in the best interest of the institution or their own best interest. This is a common local expert phenomenon not limited to HIT. When this occurs, it can sometimes be mitigated by bringing in an outside consultant (from more than 50 miles away is suggested by "common" wisdom). When the disinterested outside expert provides advice similar to the local expert, it may help improve local trust and recognition.

 Lessons Learned

- The individuals with the most expertise in IT are not always the ones making the important IT decisions.

- Organizations must have clearly defined strategic goals and tactical objectives that are conducive to the success of broad HIT initiatives.

- Informaticists should carefully evaluate the culture of an organization when considering employment.

- Poorly led or poorly designed HIT initiatives can have broad and deep negative impacts across a health system.

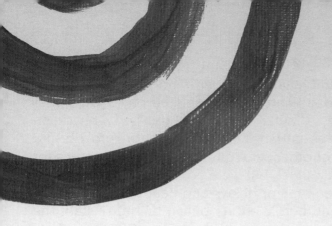

CHAPTER

20

Shortsighted Vision: CPOE after Go-Live

Editor: Christopher Corbit

Key Words:
CPOE, leadership, transformational event, vision

Project Categories:
inpatient electronic health record (EHR), computerized provider order entry (CPOE)

Lessons Learned Categories:
communication, leadership/governance, staffing resources

 Case Study

A small community hospital underwent implementation of computerized physician order entry (CPOE) in 2009, adding on to a major vendor electronic health record (EHR) system that had been in use for five years previously. From the start, the actual goals of the implementation were unclear. The vice president for medical affairs (VPMA) saw computerized provider order entry as a shortcut to improved safety and quality in a hospital that had problems with both. The chief information officer (CIO) saw his own worth measured in his success in implementing big projects, and saw this implementation as a means to burnish his reputation with his peers. The chief executive officer (CEO) liked to think of his institution as being cutting edge, and bringing advanced medicine to this semirural setting. CPOE and EHRs fit right in with that vision.

The hospital undertook the implementation with no external support beyond that provided by the vendor. There was no defined physician leader other than the chief medical officer (CMO). The CMO established a physician advisory governance group, but he essentially managed the entire process and personally authored the majority of order sets. Clinical goals and metrics for the project were established at the outset, but were not closely monitored.

The project was subject to several major delays and nearly failed entirely. However, thanks to long nights and heroic efforts put in by the IT staff, the CMO, the lead nurse informaticist, and volunteer physicians, CPOE was fully rolled out to all inpatient settings, and ultimately achieved a 90 percent adoption rate. The build had many flaws and imperfections, but most of the medical staff, largely made up of contracted hospitalists, consented to using the CPOE system. Others developed workarounds (such as faxing in paper orders or moving entirely to verbal orders), or left the medical staff entirely.

The CPOE project had made no provisions for postimplementation maintenance or clean up, and had no formal closure process for identification of outstanding issues. As the project team began to disintegrate, there were over 250 order sets implemented, but many had flaws, some major. Additionally, there were 20 to 30 specialty-specific order sets that were never created.

Within a few months after go-live, attention began to drift. CPOE project meetings ended, with no regular replacement. The CEO turned his attention to other "advanced medicine" initiatives. The CIO and his staff moved on to other big projects (Meaningful Use, a patient portal, an anesthesia module, and such). The CMO's governance group began to lose interest, and the meetings became thinly attended. Aside from a few medication safety metrics, no other benefits were measured or accounted for.

The CMO hired an experienced chief medical informatics officer (CMIO) about six months after go-live to take stock of the situation and take over where he had faltered. The CMIO generated a list of over 200 necessary fixes, some urgent, and over 50 order sets desperately needing revision. He reconstituted the physician governance group, and began to develop processes and procedures for EHR change requests and clinical content updates. However, the CIO would not make his staff available routinely to provide maintenance and enhancements. His focus remained on new big projects, and he neither knew nor cared about the day-to-day clinical operations of the medical center. The CEO also remained fixated on advanced medicine and never held his CIO or operational leaders accountable for the problems introduced by a CPOE system that could not be maintained.

Aside from a few pharmacy metrics, the CPOE system did little to improve quality and safety overall. Additionally, without sufficient maintenance staff available, all quality improvement initiatives became bottlenecked in the IT department. The queue of requests to improve, update, or enhance order sets grew longer and longer, and the quality of care drifted further and further from the ideal. Two years later, the original clinical goals and metrics had never been measured after implementation.

Nevertheless, the CIO (checking the box on a big project list) and the CEO ("Advanced medicine!") remained contentedly ignorant of any problems as they moved onto their next big initiatives. In their eyes, it was "mission accomplished."

 ## Author's Analysis

By many standards (including Stage 1 of Meaningful Use), this CPOE implementation succeeded wildly. The implementation was completed in a timely manner, and the hospital saw adoption rates approaching 90 percent. Many in the organization, including the CEO and CIO, would not disagree. But is the rate of adoption the only (or even the most important) metric of success?

The problem here is that CPOE was treated as a project, rather than a transformative event. Lacking vision and foresight, the organization could not see beyond the immediate implementation hurdles and failed to plan accordingly. A CPOE system requires regular maintenance and upkeep just to maintain a basic level of safety. And radical transformation of healthcare delivery to enable the best, most efficient care requires a great deal more than physicians typing their orders. Without sufficient resources devoted to improving the EHR, the organization cannot respond rapidly to clinical feedback or advance patient care through persistent application of quality improvement principles.

The hospital still suffers today from decisions made under the influence of poor leadership and inadequate governance.

 ## Editor's Commentary

At the inception of this institutional transformative endeavor, an obvious lack of leadership and focus led to this project being a clinical failure. Every major administrator responsible for this transformation had different objectives and measures of success. This included the lack of a true transformational team with only a very small core group of individuals responsible for major portions of the development. Even though by some measures the project can be considered successful, the actual users of the system endured extreme hardships in the entire process, possibly leading to poor quality of care.

In planning such a large-scale transformational event, several key steps must be taken to ensure the success of the project for all the stakeholders. One of the most important aspects, however, is a strong leadership to develop trust, earn credibility, and share their long-term strategy with absolute clarity.

Without the support of the stakeholders, any well-planned implementation will fail when there is no clear strategy from the leadership.

Transformational projects begin with the development of a long-term vision, a view of the best possible outcome that will inspire and give motivation to the stakeholders. These goals can be developed by one administrator, by the executive team, or may emerge from accumulative discussions among stakeholders. The most important factor is that the administrative team defines and shows a united front. A clear vision of the goals and clinical measurements of success are essential. With a well-defined vision, the overall plan will always be known and serve as a roadmap for critical decisions in times when the specifics of the project are being discussed. In this case, even though there was some attempt at clinical measures and goals, the author noted the lack of follow-through, which contributed to failing to meet the measured goals.

Another important aspect, in fact one that never ends, is to constantly keep all the stakeholders dedicated to the vision, which will take a lot of energy and commitment. Initially, a few people will immediately accept the vision, but many others will take some time to accept the change. Therefore, the transformational team will need to take every opportunity to educate participants on the importance of the strategy and what their involvement can achieve.

Finally, it is important to remain involved and approachable not only during the implementation, but long after the system is in use. The actions and staunch commitment of administration to keep the stakeholders engaged, especially during the difficult times that most of these types of projects always seem to have, is crucial. When the strategy is not clear, the commitment to the implementation of the vision and plan falters. The executive and transformational team must instill the highest level of commitment to the vision.

In hindsight—and you can argue from the start of this case—there was a significant lack of clear leadership and vision. An extraordinary amount of work was needed at the last minute to "successfully" implement the CPOE system, which ultimately required the CMO to do a majority of the work on order set creation and content. However, this work translated into requiring multiple workarounds developed by several members of the medical staff, with a number of these physicians leaving the medical staff altogether. Not a successful implementation in any measure for a successful transformational event.

This leads to another issue, which is compounded by the fact that no clear goals or measures of success were predetermined. The CEO and CIO felt that the project was a success, despite all the internal evidence indicating that it was not. This is due to the fact that end-user experience and feedback is typically lost due to it being filtered through several layers on its way to administration. This "telephone chain" effect typically changes the original content of frustration and failure to acceptance and success once the original information is slightly changed in each step from user to supervisor to manager to committee to director to vice president and finally to the executive team.

This case highlights the issues and frustrations of users when transformational leadership fails to develop a clear strategy and appropriate methods to measure achievement of goals. When this happens, the end-users, and ultimately patients, suffer. The executive team must develop a cohesive plan and vision for any large project of this size and make sure that they have the skills and ability to implement a large-scale institutional transformational event.

 Lessons Learned

- Institutional transformation events require a clear vision and specific goals spelled out by the administration.

- Keeping all stakeholders committed to the vision is a fundamental, and ongoing, commitment.

- A well-defined vision provides a roadmap to guide decisions related to the project.

- The continued maintenance of CPOE systems is just as, if not more, important than the initial work required for implementation.

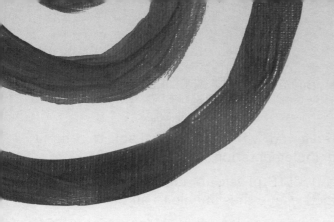

Committing Leadership Resources: A CMIO and CPOE Governance

Editor: Gail Keenan

Key Words:	Project Categories:	Lessons Learned Categories:
chief medical informatics officer (CMIO), computerized provider order entry (CPOE), executive search, leadership	inpatient electronic health record (EHR), computerized provider order entry (CPOE)	communication, leadership/governance, staffing resources

 ## Case Study

Anticipating a computerized provider order entry (CPOE) go-live within two years, a medical center decided that it needed to move beyond just a committee of physicians. The medical center had a medical informatics committee (MIC) with a chairperson. However, no physicians were involved in the day-to-day leadership of the project. Governance structure consisted of a chief information officer (CIO), with direct reports of a chief nursing informatics officer (CNIO) and a director of medical informatics. No CMIO was present due to limited budget. It was determined that a physician needed to be centrally involved with the CPOE project, with a commitment of at least seven-tenths full-time equivalents (0.7 FTE). Recruitment of the individual was as follows:

- Internal candidates were interviewed, with no individual able to commit greater than 0.25 FTE to the implementation.
- The chair of the MIC was a 0.8 FTE physician administrator (chief of medicine) and 0.2 FTE in practice, and thus unable to fill this role.
- An executive search firm was engaged to find a "physician CPOE leader."
- Candidates were screened and an individual was identified and hired for the position (0.8 FTE CPOE role, 0.2 FTE clinical practice as ambulatory care physician).
- The physician CPOE leader was to report to the director of medical informatics (nonclinician).
- The physician CPOE leader had no formal reporting relationship within the clinical governance of the medical center.
- Responsibilities of the physician included providing physician input on CPOE design and build, assisting with the MIC, and establishing liaison relationships between clinical departments and IT.

As the build progressed, the physician's importance to the project grew, mainly due to this individual's ability to gather physician input and inform the CPOE build. Soon this individual was overwhelmed with managing physician requests for the build, managing MIC meetings, and being an ambassador to the physician community in addition to the 0.2 FTE clinical practice as an ambulatory physician.

Due to this individual's lack of bandwidth and the inability of the medical center to support a CMIO role, the physician leader of sixteen months left to become a CMIO at another organization. The medical center was left with a large void, at both the project level and within the physician community. The CPOE project team sought to fill this void with two physicians who were able to contribute at 0.4 FTE each. The CNIO was able to step in and manage physicians, but only to a limited degree.

As a result of the fragmented leadership, there were project delays (including a several month delay of the CPOE go-live), a failed effort to standardize order sets, disparate physician communications, and chaotic MIC meetings. This organization has since retained physicians to assist with IT build optimization and hired a full-time CMIO.

Author's Analysis

The medical center's vision that a "project physician" could achieve success was shortsighted, in that physician input was required at two key levels—CPOE system design and build and physician "ambassador" duties. The project physician could not successfully focus on developing leadership relationships, communicating with physicians, and addressing cross-departmental issues without significant hospital support. Additionally, the physician struggled to provide sufficient input for the CPOE design and build. Both roles were full-time jobs and should not have been combined into one position. Having the project physician report to IT, rather than clinical leadership, further contributed to these problems because the project leadership (IT) lacked the management authority to address these challenges. The physician similarly underestimated the level of effort the role would take. The senior hospital management also did not effectively monitor the CPOE initiative and did not identify the evolving limits to the physician leadership for the project or address them. The MIC, as a leadership bridge for IT and clinical departments, should have served as another opportunity to identify the developing problems with the project, but that also would have required leadership accountable to the success of the CPOE project. Ultimately, the investment in the physician was lost when these bandwidth issues collided with the lack of medical center support for a CMIO.

 Editor's Commentary

The author provided an example of the costly consequences of an organization's failure to take the long view on the infrastructure and leadership needed to support health information technology (HIT). As so many others have found when there is no clear vision for HIT within one's organization, poor decisions will occur due the absence of a framework to guide effective decision making. The case suggests that the organization's leadership was not mindful of the factors associated with effective implementation of CPOE and also made no attempt to learn about the factors.

Though HIT failures can be instructive to those involved, the costs are sufficiently steep to warrant thoughtful planning and a search for feasible strategies that enhance decision making and minimize failure whenever possible. As was seen here, the management of an HIT project in isolation from an overall plan was a recipe for failure. It is in the interest of each healthcare organization to create an overall HIT vision and roadmap for achieving it that is updated at least annually. The vision and roadmap provide the basis for making sound decisions that link to the overall needs and HIT goals of the organization. As each new HIT-related problem arises, a solution can be devised that builds on the roadmap and knowledge gained through pursuing it.

In this case, the decision to hire the "physician CPOE leader" was a conclusion reached by a team anxious to see day-to-day physician leadership involvement on the CPOE project. The title of the position and job specifications suggested a short-term solution. Additionally, the combination of the narrow job scope, the physician leader being new to the organization, and the absence of formal ties to the clinical governance infrastructure made this position untenable. Ultimately, the new physician leader was beholden to multiple bosses and could not effectively carry out the role. Thus it was no surprise to learn that the physician hired as the CPOE leader eventually moved to take on a CMIO role of greater bandwidth and administrative support outside the organization. There were clearly missed opportunities to avoid this fate during the recruitment and hiring phase. The organization used an executive search firm to help fill the position but it is not clear that the expertise of the firm was used to the fullest. This type of consultant is typically paid a substantial fee to fill high-level job positions because of the consultant's specialized knowledge of the industry and talent in it. At the onset, the organization should have expected the consultant, as part of routine responsibilities, to evaluate the viability of the proposed position and present evidence-based recommendations for adjustments where needed. Had this been done, the position could have been revamped and better aligned with the organizational goals and resources before the hire. If, on the other hand, the consultant provided such feedback and it was not considered, then the organization needs to reexamine the efficacy of using costly consultant specialists whose advice is ignored.

In summary, the exorbitant costs of errors in the field of HIT suggest the need for thoughtful planning and the provision of solid evidence where possible to support decisions. This case provides a classic example of costs associated with the failure to build on existing knowledge; simply needing to recruit a new CMIO costs a significant amount of money. Even a simple review of the literature on CPOE implementation prior to designing the physician job specification could have dramatically altered the course of events in this case.

Lessons Learned

- Empower a physician leader to focus primarily on relationships, communication, and cross-departmental issues.

- Physician involvement at a project design and build level is important and time-consuming.

- Physician leaders require accountability to the clinical core of the organization.

- A medical informatics committee should continue in perpetuity and requires physician(s) to act as a bridge between clinical and IT departments.

Part II
Ambulatory Care Focus

The EHR Spotlight

Even if we had abandoned the entire implementation on the day of go-live, our institution would still be a far better place. By selecting, developing, and implementing an EHR we examined almost every part the organization. The EHR initiative shined a "spotlight" on every process, workflow, stakeholder, type of clinician, and piece of content in the entire institution and helped us understand our current state as well as develop a vision of the future.

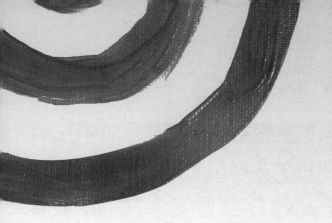

22

All Automation Isn't Good: CPOE and Order Sets

Editor: Pam Charney

Key Words:	Project Categories:	Lessons Learned Categories:
CPOE, cost, Health Level 7 (HL7), interface, laboratory, order sets, physician informaticist, results management	ambulatory electronic health record (EHR), computerized provider order entry (CPOE), laboratory information systems	data model, staffing resources, system configuration, workflow

 Case Study

An ambulatory care center was baffled by rising laboratory costs and erroneous laboratory test results. The center had hoped implementing an electronic interface between its electronic health record (EHR) and its off-site laboratory would decrease costs and errors. However, even after the implementation of the EHR the center found that costs and errors were growing each day.

After implementing the laboratory interface, the ambulatory care center hired a physician informaticist to assist. The physician soon discovered many errors in the setup of the EHR orders screen and the lab interface mapping. Table 22.1 illustrates some of these errors.

Table 22.1. Labs ordered in EHR, tests mapped in lab interface, and lab results received

Name of Order in EHR (what the clinician sees)	Name of Corresponding Test Mapped in Lab Interface (what the lab runs)	Name of Lab Result Label Mapped in HL7 Messages (what the EHR saves for clinician to see)
CPK (Creatine Kinase)	Cockroach IgE	Creatinine
Chem Screen *Note: Providers thought this was "Basic Metabolic / Chem7."	Panel of tests including amylase, CBC, CD3, CD4, glucose, urea nitrogen, cholesterol, HDL, LDL, triglycerides, alkaline phosphatase, GGT, AST, ALT, LDH	Corresponding test results
GC Probe *Note: Specimen kit at this clinic is for RNA test.	Gonorrhea RNA	Gonorrhea DNA
HIV-1/2 Antibody	HIV-1/2 Antibody	HIV-2 *Note: The HIV-2 strain is very rare in the United States.
Hepatitis C Antibody	Hepatitis C Viral Load	(not mapped; results were faxed)

These examples illustrate that lab test results the clinicians received were not what they expected when ordering the tests. Because of the errors in the laboratory interface setup, EHR orders caused thousands of automated errors leading to significant frustration for clinicians and the diagnostic laboratory company due to

- Unmet expectations
- Wasted time trying to look for the "correct" results
- Uninformed or misinformed clinical decision making
- Patient safety and risk management
- Unmet quality outcomes and pay-for-performance targets
- Unreliable data integrity of EHR results
- Costs of incorrect or unnecessary laboratory tests

To make matters worse, the prior nonclinical EHR specialist set up disease-specific panels of tests with the intention of making it easier for clinicians to quickly order tests—but this resulted in the clinicians being able to quickly order the wrong tests.

For example, there was a prenatal laboratory panel that clinicians would order with one click at every prenatal visit (CBC + UrCult + RPR + Rub + ABO + Rh + HgBE + Lead + HBsAG / ABS + HCV). However, this panel was redundant to order at every pregnancy stage and was missing critical tests at specific gestational ages as recommended by obstetrics practice guidelines. Therefore, the missing tests either were not ordered, or the clinicians had to hunt through the EHR orders screen to find those specific tests.

Another example of systematizing poor quality and high cost care is a previous HIV laboratory panel that was frequently ordered for HIV patients: the "Chem Screen" described in table 22.1 above plus "HSVIgG + HepC + HBsAG + RPR + HIVAbw / WB." In this example, not only were some tests redundant and some tests missing, but also the Hepatitis C screening test was erroneously mapped to the very expensive Hepatitis C viral load test that would not be clinically indicated for patients without Hepatitis C. One also wonders why an HIV antibody test would be repeatedly checked on known HIV+ patients.

The physician informaticist decided to tackle these laboratory order and result problems with a systematic approach instead of ad hoc troubleshooting for the following reasons:

- She recognized the profound impact these errors could have on patient safety, care quality, and operating costs.
- There were numerous errors discovered in every step of the laboratory order process:
  - Incorrect test and panel options listed in EHR
  - Incorrect mapping of orders to laboratory interface
  - Incorrect mapping of laboratory result HL7 messages into the EHR database

The physician informaticist researched which laboratory tests ought to be orderable in the EHR based on the following:

- Analyzing reports of prior utilization of laboratory tests—how often was each EHR order selected by clinicians in the past year?
- Reviewing medical evidence-based guidelines (such as recommended tests for prenatal or HIV care); these were used to create new order sets instead of current panels that were not clinically useful.

- Reviewing quality measures including the managed care Healthcare Effectiveness Data and Information Set (HEDIS) and Meaningful Use metrics about hemoglobin A1c, creatinine, and drug monitoring.

- Conducting focus groups with the ambulatory care center clinicians to build consensus around which core laboratory tests must be included in the EHR orders.

- Weighing the cost of each test against the potential benefits to clinical decision making. For example, in the previous laboratory orders setup, more than half of the available EHR orders were obscure immunoglobulin E (IgE) tests for uncommon allergens. Not only were these very expensive and often not covered by the patients' health insurance, but also these tests were rarely ordered and would be more appropriate for complex allergy patients referred to outside allergy specialists.

The physician informaticist analyzed prior data about EHR laboratory orders and results, followed by remapping all the orders and results that the ambulatory care center was planning to include in the EHR:

- For every EHR order that a clinician can select, the physician informaticist had to check that the message the interface software sends to the laboratory company has the instructions for the clinically equivalent test (that is, if a clinician orders "CPK" in the EHR, the interface map needs to tell the laboratory company to perform the test called "Creatine Kinase").

- For every incoming HL7 results message, a lab data map was created to tell the EHR where to save the result. For example, for an incoming "positive" result for HIV-1/2, the EHR needs to be set up to save that to the field with the label "HIV-1/2" instead of erroneously saving it to the "HIV-2" field or "HSV" field.

The physician informaticist also found several laboratory tests that were performed at the ambulatory care center. Instead of mapping those tests to the laboratory company, she researched and mapped the corresponding CPT codes to the EHR orders to automate billing.

By removing the clinically problematic panels and remapping the EHR-laboratory interface, the physician informaticist empowered the clinicians to provide safer and more efficient care at substantially lower costs. The resulting order screen appears in figure 22.1.

Figure 22.1. Resulting order screen

HIV Labs		HIV Initial (plus above)
☐ **HIV Quarterly**		☐ HIV-1 GENOTYPE (NY)
☐ Comprehensive Metabolic Panel		☐ Hepatitis A Ab (total)
☐ CD4 / CD8 + CBC		☐ Hepatitis B Core Ab
☐ HIV-1 RNA,QN,RT-PCR		☐ Hepatitis B Surface Ab QL
☐ **HIV Annual (plus above)**		☐ Hepatitis B Surface Ag
☐ Lipid Panel (Chol + Trig)		☐ Hepatitis C Ab EIA
☐ RPR serology		☐ CMV Ab IgG
☐ Gonorrhea + Chlamydia URINE (Aptima)		☐ Toxoplasma IgG
☐ Urinalysis (UA + Microscopy)		☐ PPD/TUBERCULOSIS ID

Provider feedback: *"This is awesome, so much easier than clicking around. It was well worth it!!!"*

 ## Author's Analysis

The above story illustrates several notable lessons. While electronic automation of processes can increase efficiency, in this case it also quickly multiplied errors with serious clinical, operational, and financial consequences. The ambulatory care center created automated processes without a qualified subject matter expert(s). As a result, the CPOE project lacked a leader with the ability to thoughtfully plan and monitor what was automated resulting in significant data integration errors ("garbage in, garbage out"). Fortunately, a physician informaticist was recruited who supplied critical expertise in the following domains:

- Current clinical knowledge about a broad range of laboratory tests used by multiple specialties (previous mapping was done by a nonclinician)

- Knowledge of evidence-based medicine guidelines and the ability to identify conflicting suboptimal practice patterns (previous panels were created by clinicians based on personal practices instead of evidence about which tests have high clinical utility)

- Expertise in EHR table structures, EHR database queries, large spreadsheets, and HL7 messaging (the prior clinical lead assisting the nonclinical EHR specialist did not understand the implications of interface mapping)

- Utilization and cost consciousness in making decisions about EHR options
- Coding, revenue cycle, and managed care incentives knowledge to bridge the gap between clinical operations and finance
- Policy and legal knowledge (such as whether federal initiatives prefer certain tests, or whether state regulations require special consent to order certain tests)
- Interpersonal and leadership skills to collaborate with the clinicians, technical staff, and laboratory company representatives
- Big picture vision that appreciated the enormous impact of system changes, while being detail oriented to troubleshoot and resolve specific problems

In short, because nearly all health IT projects automate processes at some level, it is imperative to involve physician informaticists with strong clinical, technical, financial, policy, and leadership skills.

 Editor's Commentary

The ultimate goal of healthcare information technology is to support safe, high-quality, cost-effective patient care. Any EHR should make it easy for the clinician to do the right thing, for the right patient, at the right time. Clinicians at the ambulatory care center discovered quickly that creation of the interface between the clinic and the laboratory made doing the right thing more difficult.

The problems faced by the ambulatory care center illustrate that seamless integration of data between organizations is often easier said than done. Several mistakes were made along the way—had a physician informaticist been involved from the beginning these errors could have been prevented. However, all too often individuals who have responsibility for making decisions regarding health information technology do not ensure that the right individuals are involved at each step of the process.

The ambulatory care center's new lab interface created a situation where errors in transmission of lab orders and results could have led to significant risk for patients. Table 22.1 illustrates just a few of the inconsistencies between tests ordered by providers, what was transmitted to the lab, and how results were sent back to providers. It is apparent that the lab interface system was not appropriately tested prior to use by providers.

It also appears that end-users were not included in development of the order interface. Most likely the initial order sets were created based on the thought that providers order tests depending on the patient's diagnosis. The initial order sets appear to simply have been lists of any and all tests that might be ordered for a given diagnosis without thought to provider experience, evidence supporting use of the test, or cost of the tests. Including a consultant who had domain expertise in medical informatics as well as experience as a clinician improved the usability and safety of the system. The physician informaticist revised lab order sets to fit provider workflow while adhering to the tenets of evidence-based practice, ensuring cost-effective care. Thorough mapping of the laboratory test names and testing of the system vastly improved patient safety.

Inclusion of a medical informatics expert during planning, building, and implementation of the new lab interface would most likely have prevented many of the problems that were experienced. In addition to understanding the complexity of healthcare information exchange, an expert in medical informatics would have ensured that appropriate testing of the system would have been done prior to use in a clinical setting.

 Lessons Learned

- Automation of processes can multiply errors with serious consequences.
- Qualified subject matter experts must be involved in complex process automation.
- Accurate mapping of data is critical for many healthcare processes and necessary to avoid potentially dangerous and costly errors.
- Physician informaticists must draw upon expertise in workflow, evidence-based practices, regulatory oversight, leadership, consensus building, and other areas.

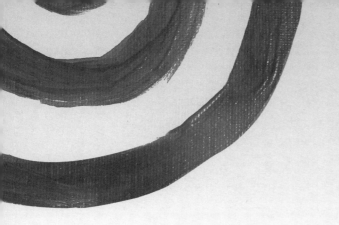

CHAPTER 23

Clinician Adoption: Community-Based EHR

Editor: Larry Ozeran

Key Words:	**Project Categories:**	**Lessons Learned Categories:**
communication, end-user training, organizational change, human-computer interaction, implementation, primary care, workflow	ambulatory electronic health record (EHR), computerized provider order entry (CPOE)	communication, leadership/governance, technology problems, training, workflow

 ## Case Study

Integration of computer-based patient records has recently been initiated in our region involving the entire infrastructure for patient-related data management and interconnecting previously isolated systems. In order to address this issue, a county council is in the process of implementing an EHR that will allow primary healthcare centers (PHCs), hospitals, and pharmacies to be integrated and able to exchange patient information. The system provides an infrastructure for sharing patient data and information between all care providers in the healthcare area. The system consists of three parts: drug information, which consists of information about all of the patients' medications and prescription-support functions, and is used to send electronic prescriptions; care documentation, which consists of all patient notes from physicians, nurses, and physical therapists; and care administration, which consists of all administrative information about the patient, such as referral handling, time booking, and registration.

During our first attempt to introduce the system in one PHC we faced the following problems:

- Absence of knowledge and skills to use the new system
- Unwillingness to adapt to the new system
- Suboptimal human-computer interaction

The lack of knowledge and skills was reported by the end-users of the system as a direct consequence of inadequate training before the system was implemented. Practitioners in general found that they did not have enough time to train before "having to do it in reality." Nurses and other nonphysician staff were particularly dissatisfied, because they thought that the training sessions were based mostly on physicians' needs.

The users also indicated that once the system went live, ongoing support was reported to be inadequate for the success of the newly implemented system. The users wanted ongoing help in order to overcome day-to-day problems.

The human-computer interaction had several technical shortcomings that remained after the implementation of the integrated system. The login process was found to be time consuming. Several features were perceived to be less than user-friendly, causing dissatisfaction and discord. Requesting a specific file consumed more time than in the previous system. The integrated system also required use of new terms, concepts, and connotations, and the users emphasized that learning this information took time.

The fact that the new system changed current workflows occasioned an unwillingness to adapt to the new system in use. The clinical personnel expressed dissatisfaction and criticism. The respondents also complained about the short timeframe for the implementation at the pilot site. They believed that the decision makers implemented the system too quickly, which caused many educational problems, mainly learning terms and navigation routines. Users questioned whether there was a strong foundation prior to implementation, including adequate staff and financial resources.

 ## Author's Analysis

Because of the high costs associated with EHRs, organizations need to have a long-term financial plan and understand the total cost of EHRs. Based on user expectations and attitudes, greater user involvement during the design and implementation phase of the system would provide better insight into existing workflows and work practices. From the users' point of view, this would have helped define the system requirements in more detail and allowed them to revise work practices to better integrate the new system.

The results of this attempted EHR implementation show that one of the most important factors that influence the outcome of integrated EHR implementation is the design of the user training program. Our users' experience of being unable to manage interaction with the new system caused secondary issues, such as the opinion that the integrated EHR was not appropriately designed. Further, it seems to be necessary to stimulate close coordination of operations where the clinical and the informatics groups work together.

The consequences of this process suggest that medical informaticians must learn from the past in order to communicate and adapt our own practices based on experience and research. However, an alternative explanation of the findings is that the unsatisfactory situation was caused by traditionally structured educational programs that were used with a new generation of technologies and end-users. Compared to a decade ago, end-users currently have more experience using computers, which means that requests and preferences should be considered. It may therefore be a mistake to believe that the training task is finished when a clinician has undergone initial training and is using the EHR. Ongoing and continued education and training may be necessary to optimize clinician efficiency and effectiveness.

How to solve the remaining technical issues is therefore not the only question when continuing the implementation of the integrated EHR. In fact, perhaps the most important question concerns how the implementation process can be adapted to meet different professional needs.

Previous evaluation studies have shown that the implementation process of a new EHR is an expensive activity. Evaluations of EHR implementations have often shown limited success, and they have failed to consistently demonstrate improvements in patient care, operating costs savings, and improvements in productivity. This study shows that we have in fact not learned from the past. The same results have been reported by hundreds of other evaluators. It seems therefore that before we continue to use the scarce resources available in healthcare organizations, it is necessary to develop strategies to involve end-users of the new system and ask them for help to accelerate organizational change as well as work routines.

Acceptance of planned change seems to be fundamental for success. Decision makers in the future should therefore plan to expedite the social process of trial and error in order to help organizations develop the necessary changes that match new technology or innovations to facilitate and accelerate the benefits that innovations have the potential to produce.

Editor's Commentary

The authors of this story are aware of this common process failure, and yet they did it anyway (or perhaps the health system's management did). Is your organization aware and still implementing the same wrong processes? If you want to save time and money, stop repeating the well-known mistakes of others! Every editor on this book has seen this process failure at least once.

You have a choice: you can ignore the needs of your users and implement what you think they need, what you want them to have, the cheapest available solution, or any number of wrong answers.

Conversely, you can work with your users. This often costs more up front and takes longer to implement, but it is cheaper in the long run and the only way to obtain a functional system.

The short version of what works follows:

1. Ensure all stakeholders are involved in the HIT selection process either directly, if your organization is small, or indirectly through representatives who have similar roles. When stakeholders are to be represented, let the stakeholders choose their representative to ensure that this person is someone who the stakeholders respect and to whom they will be comfortable presenting their perspectives. During the process, ensure that bidirectional communication is occurring—that the representatives are both sending progress reports back to their constituents and that perspectives of the constituents are being presented. This may require periodically checking in with random stakeholders who are not representatives to be certain that this communication is actually occurring.

2. Document existing workflows and how they might change under a new system. Perform a gap analysis, determining the difference between where you are and where you would like to be. Educate stakeholders about what is possible, what is affordable, and what is likely. Obtain adequate input about stakeholder priorities to ensure that the highest priorities are implemented and be prepared to explain why other priorities cannot be implemented or when they might be implemented in the future. Minimize changes to workflow.

3. Plan adequately for the implementation and training. Ensure that there is adequate staff for the expected productivity loss or, if possible in your environment, decrease the workload. Ensure that trainers are present and readily available on site initially and by phone or on call once the system seems to be working well. The decision as to whether the system is working well must be made by the users. Provide training in a learning laboratory prior to implementation if you want to reduce real-time

errors. Evaluate all participants with a standardized series of tasks before graduating them from the learning laboratory.

4. When possible, implement in phases. Lessons learned from initial implementations may then be used during subsequent phases. If you plan adequately for a phased implementation, you may be able to negotiate lower initial costs that ramp up only as you add active users. You may also need fewer extra staff to manage the initial productivity hit.

5. Include RFIs and RFPs received from your vendor as addenda in your contract to ensure the vendor meets all of their verbal commitments. Ensure that you contract for adequate training and support—this is often underestimated or underbudgeted. If you want to reduce vendor problems, include specific but reasonable penalties for noncompliance. If timelines are included, there should be clear penalties for delays.

Remember that the fastest and easiest way to go forward is for the CIO to choose the systems and implement them with no input. If you are choosing an easy path in implementing your EHR, you are probably doing it wrong. It's your choice. Choose wisely.

 Lessons Learned

- Involve clinicians in the project strategy and plan.
- Involve clinicians in the product selection process.
- Involve clinicians in implementation and management.
- Communicate effectively across all involved disciplines throughout the project life cycle.
- Effective change management and training are essential for successful EHR projects.

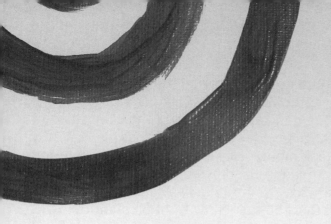

CHAPTER 24

Start Simple...Maybe: Rolling Out an EHR in a Multispecialty Group Practice

Editor: Eric Poon

Key Terms:	Project Categories:	Lessons Learned Categories:
customization, EHR, group practice, implementation, standardization, workaround	ambulatory electronic health record (EHR)	implementation approaches, system configuration

 ## Case Study

The planning and oversight of a comprehensive electronic health record (EHR) implementation at a multispecialty academic medical group practice with 40 clinics, 1,000 physicians, and 2,000 other personnel was daunting. Which practice site should go live first? How long will each clinic's go-live take? Do we install a simple system first and add the "bells and whistles" later? How should rollout staff support both practices that have gone live and practices currently going live?

The authors of this case led a two-year EHR rollout in the group practice arm of a large academic health center. This implementation represented the health center's first venture into EHRs; up until this point both the group practice's and affiliate hospital's clinical information systems were largely paper-based.

This case describes the post-EHR acquisition period in which leadership developed and executed a strategy for rolling out the EHR across its 40 clinic locations. The practice's size and the geographic spread of the clinics necessitated an EHR rollout that was staggered over time. The rollout plan initially called for bringing one clinic live each month. However, once implementation began, this timeline and the project plan were adjusted multiple times due to unexpected issues and lessons learned.

Practice leadership determined that the first clinic to implement the EHR would be a small family practice location that was geographically isolated from other primary care and specialty clinics in the group. The rationale was that the practice was not as complex as other sites. Patient volumes were relatively low, and clinic workflows were fewer and less variable. A small number of providers staffed the clinic, and the site did not participate in resident or fellow training. The expectation was that the implementation staff, including IT builders, trainers, and managers, would obtain valuable yet manageable experience with a simple implementation and use that as a springboard for the more complex clinics that remained. Moreover, if the first clinic's experience was a bad one, its relative isolation from the rest of the group would minimize the spread of negative opinions about the project to staff at other clinics. Using this same rationale of relative simplicity, the next EHR go-lives were scheduled for a residency family practice clinic and then a pediatric primary care clinic, with more complex specialty clinics to follow.

A second major decision in the clinic-by-clinic rollout was the extent to which each clinic's EHR functionality should be modified from the vendor's "model" system. This was particularly a concern in the early stages of implementation when there was tension between providing the clinics with immediately useful systems that met their expectations and moving through each location's implementation in a timely manner. On one hand, there were features of the model system that did not align well with the work processes of a given clinic or the group practice as a whole. Insufficient system customization resulted in poor acceptance of the EHR by physicians and staff. On the other hand, extensive customization at some clinics strained the capacity of the IT staff and reduced their ability to prepare the EHR for on-time rollout at upcoming clinics on the schedule. Moreover, excessive customization limited the opportunity to accomplish needed standardization of workflow and processes across clinic sites.

The implementation in the first clinic went well but a number of problems arose as the EHR rollout progressed. The implementation team struggled and user complaints increased as the EHR was installed in more complex practices, which, unlike the first practice, had resident physicians, rotating attending physicians who spent a minority of their time in clinic settings, incoming referrals, and more specialized care processes. Seemingly straightforward EHR system customizations were necessitated, such as the ability for a single provider to write prescriptions from multiple clinic locations. However, attempts to modify the model system's prescribing functionalities led to unintended malfunctions in other parts of the system that demanded significant time from IT staff and delayed the scheduled rollouts to other clinics. In such cases, where software-based solutions failed, the affected clinic's staff was forced to use unwieldy workarounds. By the time the final clinic's EHR was installed, the rollout schedule had been delayed multiple times, and the practice was planning for a new round of system customizations to address many problems that arose but went unsolved during the initial implementations.

 Author's Analysis

Leading an EHR rollout in a group practice provided many lessons. Implementing a complex system that significantly changes care delivery processes may never be perfectly predictable, but there were two decisions in particular that we would have handled differently.

First, we would have chosen a more representative clinic for the first EHR go-live. Because the first clinic was the simplest, our implementation team developed a biased understanding of the implementation process. The team spent a significant amount of time preparing for the first go-live, and this created inertia that led them to force-fit solutions that did not work in more complex clinics. The decisions made for a basic primary care clinic did not translate to a complicated surgical practice. Because it was difficult to revise decisions and modify team member behavior on the fly, the more complicated needs of other practices were often accomplished using workarounds.

A better approach would have been to begin our rollout with a clinic that was maximally representative of our practice's processes, such as resident training and incoming referrals. One of our ear, nose, and throat (ENT) clinics, which is moderately complex, has significant procedural activity, and serves as both a physician referral and direct patient referral practice may have provided a better starting point. This strategy would have exposed our team to an initial set of experiences that would better generalize to future implementations. Further, our training and build decisions would have been more representative of the practice as a whole, likely necessitating fewer workarounds.

Another potential improvement was our approach to customizing the vendor's model EHR system. A model system's functions are designed to work for the "average" patient, which ultimately means that it works for very few specific patients. However, our attempts to customize the EHR focused extensively on each clinic's idiosyncratic workflows. We failed to use our limited customization time and resources on solutions that would transcend the entire practice. Consequently, we failed to achieve key workflow standardizations that could have improved the efficiency and quality of care. Tasks such as attending physicians' documentation in resident notes, effective communication with referring physicians, and the movement of patients and information between the practice and our hospital partner were not accomplished as expertly as possible. A better approach to the initial customization of our EHR would have been to identify and customize such practice-wide workflows. Instead, we focused first on each clinic's microsystem, which merely achieved clinic-level standardization on tasks that likely had lower overall value.

 ## Editor's Commentary

This case calls to attention the different approaches EHR implementations could take. When the EHR technology is relatively immature and the outcome of its implementation uncertain, it is reasonable to start small and learn from early mistakes before scaling up the implementation to the rest of the healthcare organization. However, there is often a price to pay with this incremental strategy. First, the experience of early adopters of the EHR technology may exert disproportionate influence over its customization or ongoing development. If the needs of the early adopters differ from the rest of the larger organization, the resulting design could be less than optimal. The authors of the case stated that they wished they had started implementation at a more "representative" practice. That sentiment is understandable, but if workflow patterns have historically been developed organically in a parochial way in different practice settings, one has to ask whether a truly representative practice exists. Second, the incremental implementation strategy often serves to perpetuate the patchwork of idiosyncratic workflows, and deprives the healthcare organization the opportunity to design in a rational way a healthcare delivery system that truly serves the needs of its patient population.

One trend that is emerging with EHR implementations calls for design sessions up front that involve key stakeholders from the entire organization. This approach, which typically requires significant participation by both clinical leaders and front-line clinicians, encourages clinicians to think beyond the practice habits they have developed over the years at the local practice level and consider new approaches. During these sessions, critical issues such as interpractice communication, multidisciplinary care, transitions of care across different settings, patient and family engagement, and clinical performance improvement inform the group's thinking. If successfully executed, they offer the organization an opportunity to leverage the EHR implementation to optimize workflow and remove inefficiencies.

However, this comprehensive and inclusive approach to EHR customization and design brings its own risks. These design sessions can become unwieldy and unproductive if they are not well facilitated by those who understand the functionality of the EHR, its limitations, and different ways it could be used in different clinical settings. They also require the clinical participants to have a mature understanding of the goals of EHR implementation and what they can realistically expect out of an EHR. If the organization does not have the capacity to make design decisions quickly, or if the organization becomes overly ambitious by addressing too many clinical processes, these sessions can fail. In short, the comprehensive and inclusive design approach requires a fine balancing act.

Clearly, certain situations call for the incremental approach and others call for a more comprehensive and inclusive one. As the EHR implementation experience broadens, one might expect a growing evidence base to inform future choices. Unfortunately, the EHR implementation experience (either positive or negative) is not well published, and often remains proprietary knowledge for the EHR companies or implementation consultants. A national registry to track EHR implementation successes and failures would help advance the science of EHR implementation, but until that is developed, we will need to rely on anecdotal cases such as this one to inform implementation decisions.

 Lessons Learned

- Implementing a complex system that significantly changes care delivery processes may never be perfectly predictable.

- Engage key stakeholders from the entire organization in design sessions.

- Evaluate an organization's needs for incremental versus comprehensive implementations to assess the risks and benefits of each approach.

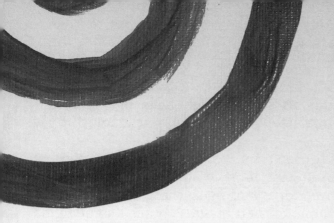

Leadership and Strategy: An Ambulatory EHR

Editor: Larry Ozeran

Key Words:	Project Categories:	Lessons Learned Categories:
electronic health record (EHR), enterprise strategy, physician champion, project management, vision	ambulatory electronic health record (EHR)	leadership/governance, project management, staffing resources

 Case Study

Whether it is your first bicycle ride, your first date, or the first step your child takes, you never forget your "first time." I will never forget my first installation of an electronic health record (EHR): it was an utter failure.

In the early 1990s, as a full-time faculty physician in infectious disease, my employer was a multihospital system in a major metropolitan area. Among many other facilities, the system operated methadone maintenance and treatment programs. We were awarded a grant to provide primary human immunodeficiency virus (HIV) care to former substance users in the inner city, a public-private initiative to improve healthcare to one especially underserved focus of the HIV epidemic.

As medical director for the grant programs, collecting and reporting grant-required specifications was my job. We provided a standard of care reflecting the best evidence-based medicine at the time: HIV monitoring (CD4 counts), antiretroviral therapy, prophylaxis to prevent opportunistic infection, screening and treatment for tuberculosis, screening for chlamydia and gonorrhea, periodic Pap smears, and mental health assessment were among the key standards tracked for the grant.

We deployed the most commonly used technology for clinical data capture at the time: paper forms. Despite our best efforts, data discrepancies began to appear. Patients sometimes arrived for urgent visits when their charts were elsewhere. Medication refills by phone created progress notes and addenda that were not always collated with the chart in a timely fashion.

Our wonderful paper forms did not always reflect the degree of care provided. No matter how many check boxes we had, how complete the requested data set, or how bright the color of paper, many staff would not update the paper form completely each and every time. It came to pass that I would scour each chart every month to monitor compliance. It was not only time-consuming but I sensed that even with my best efforts a key datum might escape my notice in the growing number of paper charts and forms.

It seemed that an EHR could capture medications, CD4 counts, and conditions during the course of care, obviating the need for duplicate data entry on a data collection form. The EHR could manage a list of medications and print out prescriptions as needed. An ongoing problem list could be maintained. Simple queries could generate performance reports. Missing paper charts would be but distant memories of the past.

We had no formal software process. With the quality committee's approval, we sought software and hardware for an EHR with our grant renewal application. Once funding was approved, we simply selected one of the better known products. As time drew near to purchase the EHR, I was confident the project would be a complete success. Our clinical team wanted the EHR. The grant sponsor approved our budget modification. What could go wrong?

For starters, the project champion would leave.

Unexpectedly, I was offered and took another job opportunity within the system. I would no longer work on the EHR project but I had a colleague who was more of a technophile than I. Confidently passing the baton to my friend, I was unaware that being a successful change agent requires skills different from a facility with technology.

With a Joint Commission hospital survey coming, I was thrown into my new position with little time to follow the new EHR project. After the Joint Commission survey, I took the opportunity to check up on my old friends in the HIV primary care program. I was surprised to learn that neither the software nor hardware was installed. The same paper-based charts that preceded my departure remained in place. Nothing had changed. What went wrong?

Author's Analysis

As someone stated before the Certifying Commission for Health Information Technology, "Adoption of an EHR is an ugly, ugly process" (Pizzi 2007), but it is not just EHR adoption. According to a 2002 report from the National Institute of Standards and Technology, up to 25 percent of commercial software projects are abandoned before completion. Project failure is not uncommon in IT inside or outside of healthcare (RTI Health, Social, and Economics Research 2002).

The literature is replete with advice on how to avoid failure. John Glaser describes critical success factors for clinical information systems that apply to our failed EHR project (Glaser 2005).

1. Strong organizational vision and strategy.

2. Talented and committed leadership.

3. A partnership between the clinical, administrative, and information technology (IT) staffs.

4. Excellent implementation skills, especially in project management and support.

Although my section chief and department chair gave formal approval to the EHR project and the colleague replacing me as project champion agreed with my personal vision, there was no enterprise EHR strategy.

The project was conceived and submitted without the knowledge, advice, or consent of our IT staff. They learned of the project only after its approval.

No one on our EHR team had IT project management experience. Without project management expertise, any IT project is at risk.

After 10 years of informatics experience, I now know that the odds were against this particular ambulatory EHR project. Neither the time nor environment was right for it yet. Too many of the critical success factors were missing for it to have turned out any other way.

 ## Editor's Commentary

It is regrettably common for well-meaning, smart people to underestimate what is required to accomplish a successful IT implementation, both in and out of healthcare. In this case, some critical aspects were present: a physician champion, supportive leadership, and adequate funding. The key project faults were not clearly articulating the project's needs through a needs assessment and gap analysis before selecting products, and not involving all of the stakeholders, most notably IT staff. As a relatively isolated, focused project, having an enterprise EHR strategy may have made the project more cost effective, but probably was not necessary for the project to succeed.

Without additional details about the specifics of the environment, it is just as hard now to determine what should have been done as it was then. We do not know the number of physical locations, which staff would access the system, what authentication would be needed, and how functional privileges would be allocated. In the absence of specifics, we can only return to generic recommendations to add to those described by Glaser:

5. Identify all stakeholders, educate them about technology specific to the project, and seek their input; this does not appear to have been done for this project.

6. Clearly state what the system is to accomplish in several detailed statements; in this project, there seemed only a general outline of what was to be accomplished.

7. Compare what technology you currently have to what you need to accomplish those stated goals (your gap analysis); apparently this was not done.

8. Determine your budget (this was done) and how much of your goals you can accomplish with that money.

9. Create lists of features and functions that support your goals and use them to determine which products can best meet your needs within your budget; this does not appear to have been done.

10. Define scripts that you can follow to test the validity of vendor claims in your environment and run them against the three most likely candidates; there does not appear to have been any due diligence done for the vendor selling the product selected or a comparison of the project needs to the product selected or to any other products for that matter.

Had these issues been addressed in addition to the positive factors that were accomplished (for example, having an effective physician champion, adequate funding, supportive leadership), the project would have been much more likely to succeed.

 Lessons Learned

- Articulate a clear project (and enterprise) strategy and project plan including timeline and desired outcomes.

- Perform a needs assessment prior to product selection.
- Involve all stakeholders in the decision-making process, including clinicians, administrators, IT staff, and anyone else who may "touch" the planned system; administrative support is critical.
- Evaluate several products or solutions with tests comparable to use in your actual environment.

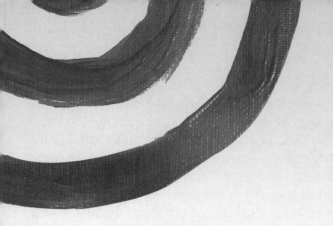

Designing Custom Software for Quality Reports: A Community Health Center's EHR

Editor: Brian Gugerty

Key Words:	Project Categories:	Lessons Learned Categories:
ambulatory electronic health record (EHR), database structure, data mining, disease management, primary care, quality improvement, scope	ambulatory electronic health record (EHR)	data model, project management

 ## Case Study

Our federally qualified health center (FQHC) wanted an EHR that would allow aggregate analysis of care and streamline encounter billing. In 1996, there were very few good, affordable EHRs appropriate for a small practice, so "the deciders" hired a young, ambitious software programmer and we four primary care nurse practitioners consulted in the design of a clinical and billing program that was to be for in-house use only. The programmer assured everyone that he could do the work in about six months! Over the next four years, in addition to maintaining the volume of patient care, we analyzed workflow, selected data to be captured, classified data elements as to coding systems and relationships, and iteratively tested the developing EHR. The program was written in structured query language (SQL) with open database connectivity (ODBC). We emphasized to the programmer that, in order to use the data for quality improvement, we needed structured data entry, standardized terminology, a user interface to promote consistent data entry, and a relational database that would link diagnoses, interventions, and outcomes. We were especially interested in capturing primary care interventions of patient education and case management, in addition to medications, procedures, and follow-up.

When the clinical software was ready and we went "live" to document encounters, we still could not print prescriptions, download electronic laboratory results, or trigger encounter bills. Nevertheless, the expanded programming team arranged for necessary hardware and networks, directed staff training, scheduled implementation and archival data entry, and provided technical support—when they weren't selling the software to other health centers. We went "live" all at once, in December 1999. Data were stored on a server in the main site that was accessible remotely by dial-up modem with password protection. After documenting a full six months of primary care, I received funding to study the reliability of the data for quality assessment. Quality audits that I did with a Crystal Reports expert were extremely challenging because of the lack of a data dictionary and a data table structure that had "grown like Topsy." Furthermore, the in-house programmers, who were busy marketing the software, were not available to perform quality assurance checks. The report expert had to determine by himself which of several database maps he was given actually matched the existing database structure.

The quality audits that we managed to generate revealed that diagnoses, interventions, and outcomes were not linked, much terminology was inconsistent and nonstandard, and differing data entry patterns had resulted in scrambled data storage. Therefore, we could not verify that patients with chronic illness received care according to national guidelines, or that preventive care such as cancer screening was properly and promptly followed up. For example, interventions recorded for 30 patients with diabetes showed patient education that included the following information: 5 stop smoking, 3 nutrition, 4 diet, 5 exercise, 2 weight loss, 5 chronic illness, 7 diabetic care, 7 sign/symptom of illness, 12 other. Definitions for these suspiciously overlapping interventions were nonexistent. Without a laboratory interface and discrete variables for cholesterol, glycosylated hemoglobin, or urine microalbumin results, and with inconsistent data entry and database storage, aggregate data could not be retrieved. Similar issues were found for hypertensive and depressed patients seen over the period. In addition, data mining for appropriate follow-up of Pap smears was not reliable for quality assessment, because of inconsistent documentation of laboratory results and text notes of the follow-up plan.

Author's Analysis

Our lessons learned are right in line with Bakken's "five building blocks of an informatics infrastructure for evidence-based practice...":

1. Standardized terminologies and structures

2. Digital sources of evidence

3. Standards that facilitate healthcare data exchange among heterogeneous systems

4. Informatics processes that support the acquisition and application of evidence to a specific clinical situation

5. Informatics competencies (Bakken 2001)

Digital sources of evidence include EHRs equipped with appropriate standardized terminologies and operated by healthcare providers who are competent in data entry. Data mining from EHRs is extremely difficult without defined, standardized terminologies. In this case, the providers were limited by insufficient knowledge of structured language and database design. The programmer had no prior experience in healthcare. Lack of agency resources reduced iterative software development and the potential for group learning. Furthermore, programming to create key labor-saving capabilities for e-prescribing, electronic download of laboratory results, guideline-based templates to remind and record orders for common encounters, automatic tracking for follow-up visits, a flow sheet of interventions given, and interface to billing was never accomplished. Nevertheless, appropriate interventions documented over six months for diabetes, hypertension, and depression did include health teaching, guidance, and counseling; case management and referral; procedures; and medications.

The resulting EHR was essentially a resource-intensive exercise in creating and implementing a rough beta version of software that worked fairly well for individual patient documentation but that was totally unacceptable for quality assessment and improvement. Much of the potential of electronic data aggregation for practice evaluation was lost in a provider focus on individual care. Although the primary care providers had each learned the research process and frequently read clinical research articles, the EHR was not seen as a tool for research and evaluation. Fundamental rules of research, such as identification and definition of key data elements, accurate data entry, and advance planning for analyses, were lost in the challenge of software development during day-to-day clinical care responsibilities. Clinical consciousness did not expand to research consciousness as the EHR developed.

Using informatics to build evidence from clinical practice has great potential to enhance our understanding of the most valuable and effective interventions in primary healthcare, in the face of expanding demand and shrinking supply of providers and payment. Furthermore, integrating decision support into documentation promises to promote "best practices" that are already known. The experience described here contributed a great deal to my own continuing education and my current involvement in efforts such as the Certification Committee for Healthcare Information Technology (CCHIT) and clinical informatics to improve public health.

 Editor's Commentary

The author states that "fundamental rules of research, such as identification and definition of key data elements, accurate data entry, and advance planning for analyses, were lost in the challenge of software development during day-to-day clinical care responsibilities." Thus, the original goals of the system, "aggregate analysis of care and streamline[d] encounter billing," were consequently and similarly "lost." The takeaway message from this case study is that if you want to make sense of data and information in an EHR on the back end, it matters a great deal how you structure and input data on the front end. The author "got" that key lesson.

For a book about lessons learned from HIT failures, the case study presented here certainly illustrates failure well. Yet we are well advised to judge historical events and figures in the context of their times, not ours. The year 1996, when this effort was begun, is a bygone historical era if measured by Internet time. Yes, the Internet was invented well before 1996, but it was not until 1997 that it began to be truly widely adopted and used. Therefore, a first reaction to judge hiring one programmer to design and build a wide-ranging and multiple-module clinical and billing information system in six months as hopelessly naïve must be resisted. Especially in ambulatory care settings, these things were still being done in, as my son calls it, "the olden days."

There is evidence of much good thinking at the beginning of this effort and throughout to attempt to incorporate fundamental principles of data structuring and clinical terminologies, but again we have come a long way in this regard since 1999 when the system went live. So I cannot fault this team except that explicitly selecting a small set of clinical terminologies and making the effort to stick to that set when and where possible might have been helpful and should have been within their scope of expertise. SNOMED, CCC (previously known as HHCC) or NIC/NOC/NANDA, and of course the old standards ICD-9 and CPT were good candidates for this project.

The software developer on this project installed alpha, or at best beta code, and effectively abandoned it to go off to sell the software elsewhere. Vendors currently cannot get away with so flagrant a violation of good business practices, yet this "old" vivid story in microcosm sometimes remains a problem with established information techonology (IT) vendors within, and beyond, healthcare. Sales are extremely important to the HIT vendor companies, as they should be, but sometimes in acquisition/sales processes that go awry, there can be significant mismatches with what the capabilities of the software are and the expectations of the customer of that software. The author's response, getting involved in the CCHIT EHR standards rather than being turned off from informatics completely, is commendable. The expertise from this early HIT initiative will be helpful to the author and many others. I would, however, caution that CCHIT accreditation may be necessary but should not be sufficient to vigorously probe the vendors and the systems that they offer during an acquisition process; acquisition processes should scrutinize the capabilities of existing HIT solutions and the expectation gap on several levels. In defense of the developer, there appears to have been significant scope creep during this project; expanding scope in both scale and complexity is common in HIT initiatives, especially as customers develop more sophisticated understanding of their own needs. Collaboration and transparent, honest communication between a vendor and customer are usually the best solutions to potential conflicts because of scope creep. A solid project plan and an experienced project manager, perhaps in the form of a third-party consultant, might have made a big difference by offering an objective viewpoint.

 Lessons Learned

- Standardized terminologies and data sets are required for aggregate reporting.
- Digital sources of information facilitate standardized data capture.
- HIT will only deliver the functionality for which it is designed (that is, an individual patient record compared with population-based reporting).
- It is rare that the complexity of an HIT initiative can be met by a single programmer.

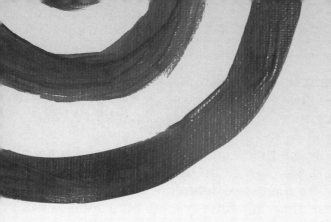

CHAPTER
27

If It's Designed and Built by One, It Will Not Serve the Needs of Many: Custom-Developed EHR

Editor: Scot Silverstein

Key Words:	Project Categories:	Lessons Learned Categories:
communication, design, development, electronic health record (EHR), stakeholder participation	inpatient electronic health record (EHR)	leadership/governance, staffing resources, workflow

 Case Study

In the late 1980s, a young resident physician at a large hospital took a year from clinical duties for research activities. One of the specialty services wanted to collect patient information on a notebook computer. With a programming background and a long-standing interest in electronic medical records, the resident thought this would be a great opportunity.

There were brief discussions about who would serve as supervising attending and what the service wanted the program to do in general, but mostly the resident was left alone to pursue the dream. After the first month, the local system was able to connect to separate radiology, dictation, and laboratory systems. The local computer would login as a user, use recursive screen scraping routines (developed by the resident) to collect and filter the data, and assign it to the correct patient. The attending was informed and seemed pleased.

During the remaining months, some time had to be spent doing other research activities, but their impact was limited on the EHR project. Being a DOS-based system, windowing options were limited, but a full screen approach was able to accept mouse clicks for cursor positioning and selection of menu items. A series of menus allowed the user to move from one patient to another, enter new patients, and pass between sections of a patient's chart.

The resident even developed a novel hierarchical encoding system for examination findings, patient complaints, anatomic regions, and so on. Two separate tools were created. One enabled authorized users to create ontologies in a hierarchical fashion that were represented in the 32-bit identifier itself, allowing data size to shrink and accelerating recovery of matching patients with direct and indirect matches for performing drug studies or other research. The other tool allowed viewing or selecting from the lists the users had created. There was no limit to the number of ontologies that could be created.

Multiple portions of the EHR came live: vital signs, a patient's daily fluid inputs/outputs with predefined fluids to pick from expandable lists, transferred data from other information systems, pick lists for patients, entry of new patients, and so on. The system was documented and one hospital employee was trained. The department purchased a notebook computer and, as far as the resident could tell, everything was working and ready to go. But was it?

When the resident physician graduated the residency program, the system had been used rarely, if at all.

 ## Author's Analysis

The system was designed with the resident's skill set and needs in mind, not those of the ultimate user(s). The system was very advanced for its time, but perhaps too complicated for the user at the time. There seemed to be inadequate input from the other users about what they truly needed and how the system would work best for them.

In the end, a great opportunity for promoting HIT was lost because of inadequate communication with the stakeholders. Even when project technologists have clinical backgrounds, they do not speak for everyone.

Editor's Commentary

This case study of a single person's efforts to create innovative HIT is a microcosm that is representative of common problems that occur in healthcare information technology (IT) design and implementation by larger groups and by vendors.

The major issue is false assumptions about the needs, enthusiasm, desire to contribute time and effort, and ultimate drivers and motivators (or demotivators, such as fear of what robust data might reveal) of HIT end-users and other stakeholders. The example is especially relevant to the creation of customized IT for focused specialty areas or for biomedical research, but also applies to unremarkable HIT such as EHR and computerized provider order entry (CPOE) facilitating clinical care delivery.

A specialty service wanted to aggregate data drawn from larger systems for varied research purposes. The needs assessment and design discussions were brief and identified just one physician who was to act as a spokesperson for a larger group. Inadequate involvement of stakeholders through inadequate interaction, as well as selection of a "representative" or representatives whose own knowledge of true needs might be inadequate, or who might emphasize their own interests over others, are common errors. These mistakes fall under the general category of underrepresentation of stakeholders. These stakeholders include users and those who are affected, or potentially affected, by the output or outcomes from information system deployment.

Introduction of new technologies often creates winners and losers in a competitive environment. Those who are left out, especially those who might perceive the technology as a threat and who are not given the opportunity to express this perception and negotiate, can become obstacles to project success (through passive or even active aggressive behaviors, for example).

This resident only explored others' needs briefly, and then was "left alone" to do things as he or she saw fit. Although IT personnel and vendors might find that situation desirable in order to complete a project within a limited time period, in the end it increases the risk of rejection and failure of the HIT project significantly. One person, even a healthcare domain expert (or worse, a nondomain expert such as a junior medical professional or a nonmedical IT professional) is an inadequate representative of the need for planning, design, acquisition, implementation, and life cycle enhancement of an HIT application. These are complex processes requiring adequate involvement of, and frequent collaboration between, IT personnel, clinical personnel, and often their management who control resources.

The medical resident (trainee) spent significant time developing an application and coding system innovative for its time. The system may have been far more advanced than other applications in use, with integrated ontology development and maintenance tools and no artificial limits on data complexity. The resident probably expected users to recognize its advanced nature and adopt it enthusiastically on the basis of its technological sophistication and elegance.

The reality was different. Few used the system, and only rarely. This was not paradoxical. Issues that could have contributed to the lack of acceptance and use, which currently remain unchanged, include the following:

- The system as designed might not actually meet the research needs of a variety of stakeholders, as design parameters were set by too few users (in this case, one).

- The designer's own assumptions may not have been correct for the situation.

- The designer may have overestimated the ability, desire, and resources available for users to learn the system and integrate it into their daily workflows.

- The system might have been excellent technically, but difficult and cryptic to those for whom it was made. Iterative and incremental development processes with involvement of a variety of end-users might yield a more satisfactory user experience.

- Only one person was trained in use of the system. There was a lack of training of others as backups or independent users. Inadequate training, in numbers and depth, is a common cause of end-user difficulty and rejection of HIT. It may have been assumed that the one employee who was trained would then pass this knowledge to others. This is not a good assumption in the complex and competitive world of biomedicine.

A major lesson that can be learned from this case is the need for adequate user and stakeholder participation in all phases of HIT design, development, and deployment. This differs from the more traditional management information systems development process, which is often done in relative isolation after an initial assessment and design phase.

Another lesson that should be learned is the need for HIT project leaders and key personnel to not allow their own biases and assumptions to color the deliverables. This will too often occur in a manner that makes sense to them from their other expertise and experience, but might create a very unsatisfactory and unproductive user experience, and a distraction from other important work, for those "in the trenches" who have to do the actual healthcare work.

Lessons Learned

- Design for the needs of end-users (clinicians) as a group.
- Involve clinicians in system design.
- Plan to integrate systems into clinicians' workflows.
- Train end-users in sufficient quantity and depth of knowledge of a technology to enable peer learning and peer support for use of HIT.

All Systems Down...What Now? Ambulatory EHR

Editor: Christopher Corbit

Key Words:	Project Categories:	Lessons Learned Categories:
ambulatory, communication, downtime, EHR, e-prescribing	ambulatory electronic health record (EHR)	communication, leadership/governance, technology problems, training

 Case Study

A large, multisite ambulatory care health system with over 50 physicians and mid-level providers implemented a market leading electronic health record (EHR). Within two years the health system is using the EHR for all clinically focused processes: patient visits are scheduled in the EHR; patients are checked in and triaged in the EHR; and clinicians document all aspects of patient care in the EHR, including communications with nurses and other colleagues about patient management. All orders are entered and managed within the EHR, such as prescriptions, diagnostic tests, and internal and external consult requests. The EHR is digitally linked to pharmacies through a statewide e-prescribing system. Additionally, the health system has leveraged problem lists and procedure codes for clinical decision support alerts that guide an individual patient's care. Outside records are either received by the EHR via direct data interfaces (that is, lab results) or entered as scanned documents. Staff use both mobile and fixed devices supported by a wireless network, depending on their workflow needs. Beyond regular office hours, providers use remote access to the EHR to help manage patients when on call. Occasionally there are problems with the system's slowness and performance, but mostly the EHR functions well and has become a critical resource to the health system. The health system has started the process to attest for Centers for Medicaid and Medicare Services (CMS) Stage 1 Meaningful Use dollars.

One morning, around 9:30 a.m., clinicians and administrative staff at a large site in the health system begin to experience EHR freezes; "hourglasses" spin on the display screen for seconds and sometimes minutes, orders "hang" before completing, and other data entry steps or data review tasks become very slow. Providers and administrative staff at the site ask each other if the problems are site-wide or just affecting a few people. After another hour they learn that everyone at the site is experiencing the same problems. A call is placed to the IT help desk. The EHR functions slowly, but is usable during patient care. As the morning progresses, the system delays worsen and providers report that the entire EHR is freezing and shutting down. One physician says he rebooted his laptop three times without any improvement. Another physician reports feeling embarrassed when a patient in an exam room asked about a recent MRI result and it took three minutes to open the MRI report. A nurse complains that it took five minutes to pick up an order for a flu vaccine and document it was given to a patient, instead of the typical one to two minutes. Two physicians discuss whether or not the site should revert to paper, but they are reluctant to do so, given that all patient information is only available in the EHR and that any data manually collected would need to be entered into the system eventually.

One local site administrator announces that due to the problems with the EHR, the site will not schedule any more patients that day because they are already two-thirds booked (which is typical for a busy morning). By 11:30 a.m., the site learns that the entire health system is being affected by the EHR performance problems. Each task a clinician enters takes up to five minutes and occasionally the entire EHR freezes, at which point the computer must be rebooted. Before 12:00 p.m., the director of information technology sends an e-mail to all staff that the health system is experiencing major problems with EHR performance and that the IT team is working with the EHR vendor to address the problems. The director of IT sympathetically notes that he "feels your pain." Another local site's providers agree that they will document all visits on paper. Prescription pads are found and distributed to providers. A nurse practitioner suggests deferring coding of visits until the system resumes normal function.

A physician notices that the next three patients to arrive have multiple, complex medical problems, take many medications, and have frequent diagnostic tests to review. He asks the patients to reschedule for another day, explaining that the EHR is down. The registration desk at the local site is instructed to inform patients as they arrive that due to problems with the computer system, only brief visits and medication refills will be provided. A nurse fields a call from a pharmacy—a physician had renewed a patient's narcotic pain medications for a much higher dose than the patient usually receives. The physician writes a new prescription and recognizes that he misunderstood the patient's reported dose, which could not be verified without the EHR. For the next few hours, physicians and nurses struggle to treat patients with diabetes, heart disease, and mental illness without access to past records, medication lists, test results, or care plans. The staff spends much of the day apologizing to patients, some of whom are angry. Most patients must reschedule to return another day.

 ## Author's Analysis

After extensive review of the problem by both the health system's IT team and the vendor, a plan was set to upgrade servers and modify database configurations that were identified as the cause of the poor performance of the EHR. The health system made several key errors that caused the downtime to be a bigger organizational problem than it had to be. The health system did not realize that with a fully implemented EHR, care could not continue "as usual" when the EHR went down. Without the EHR, providers made mistakes, potentially harming patients. Health system productivity suffered, which not only affected the organization as a whole but also could have affected the staff since all employees receive productivity based incentive compensation. Staff also felt insecure and unsupported by the organization, having felt forced to provide less than optimum care.

The health system did not have any triggers for clinician and administration leadership to make decisions about what to do at different stages of system outages, including when to revert to paper documentation, when to reschedule patients, and even when to stop providing care. Inadequate communication meant staff was not informed about problems with IT as they evolved and did not know how to respond to the problems. Lastly, the patients' response to the outage should not be overlooked—if events like this continue with any regularity at a health system, patients will likely start going elsewhere for care.

The health system should have prepared and practiced for downtime, just like fire drills are practiced in case of a fire. Without practice drills, neither clinicians nor administrators can know what to do during downtime. Downtime drills should include all aspects of downtime management, including communication protocols and paper-based documentation processes.

 ## Editor's Commentary

As electronic health records become "mission-critical" elements of patient care, downtime is an extremely disruptive process and significant issue for most patient care settings. As we move away from paper charts, there is an increasing reliance on EHR for clinical information and workflow. If not adequately planned for, downtime may be considered such a disruption in services as to threaten the safety and welfare of patients. Therefore, policies and procedural support that exemplify best practices during downtime are absolutely necessary.

Downtime may happen at anytime—even a few hours after go-live! Thus, you need to plan and test your downtime procedures at the same time you are implementing your EHR, which is not an easy task and normally overlooked by project management. In development, focus on best practices and guidelines to provide uninterrupted service in an efficient manner before, during, and after downtime.

Although a detailed plan on developing a downtime plan is beyond the scope of this discussion, presented here is a generalized framework to either begin your downtime policy and procedure creation, or to review what you already have in place and help augment it. The creating of downtime procedures can be broken down into four main categories:

1. **Provider and staff communication**: Once downtime has been identified, consistent communication is vital throughout the downtime and its recovery among all stakeholders affected by the downtime.

2. **Availability of historical clinical data**: Access to patient information by the clinical and office staff is vital to maintaining patient safety and optimal care throughout the downtime.

3. **Continuing operational activities**: Ongoing clinical care and support for business activities must be maintained within the framework of a downtime, episode as exemplified in this particular case presentation.

4. **Recovery and reconciliation of data**: After the downtime is over, the reconciliation of data back into the EHR is fundamental for continued patient safety and quality of care.

With the focus on these general areas, divide the work into discrete phases and address specific workflows (such as order entry or documentation).

Systematically tackle questions about how each group of stakeholders (physicians, nurses, office staff) responds in each downtime phase across each process, with a focus on workflow. Each group will need to specifically identify the areas where they are dependent upon the other groups for information or logistical planning.

One of the first priorities in assisting the delivery of clinical care during system downtime is providing clinicians access to historic clinical information. The downtime solution should be able to provide as much historical information as is feasible. This needs to be as up to date as possible and easy to access, or a frustrating situation can be made worse and patient safety can be further compromised. Even if you have designed and implemented your EHR backup with a near-real-time incremental update system, pieces of information may be lost. It may be possible to have a regularly scheduled extract of data including demographics, medications, problem lists, and immunizations saved to a secure computer at a defined timeframe that can be printed in the event of downtime.

There may be other sources of historical data that can be accessed outside of the EHR. For example, ancillary systems may have a direct log-on or portals that nonlab personnel can access. Also, picture archiving and communication systems (PACS) frequently store diagnostic imaging reports as well as the images internally. Transcribed reports are frequently stored in scanning or document management systems outside the integrated clinical system.

Maintaining operational activity during downtime may be one of the most difficult tasks to achieve, but if planned for accordingly and practiced (just like fire or disaster drills), the challenges can be minimized. There are several critical areas that need to be addressed in your plans, which include the clinical and office staff. Downtime forms need to be accessed quickly; these are entered later or scanned depending on the EHR or policy. Laboratory and radiology results will need to be reported on paper, as well as any standing orders held for later entry into the EHR. Also, it is imperative to have prescription pads always accessible, along with medication and allergy lists. Finally, have the most commonly used patient instructions preprinted and available to give to patients at discharge.

Another priority during downtime is providing clinicians the tools to document and implement treatment plans. Once clinicians begin using an EHR, they have a tendency to forget even deeply embedded knowledge. This can be one of the greatest hazards of EHRs. Most EHRs have clinical decision support tools built into the system. An example of this is to have specific reminders within the documentation, such as asking about influenza or pneumococcal immunization. Without being prompted by the documentation, either the physician or the nurse may not be reminded to ask this question since they are accustomed to being prompted to do so. The office staff is already working without their customary tools, so anything that can be done to simplify and make the processes more efficient is very beneficial.

When switching to paper for documentation, preprinted templates and flow sheets should maintain the same design style and embedded clinical decision support as in the EHR. With the same style as the EHR, it will be easier for the clinicians to maintain their workflow. It is important to remember that once you have your paper downtime forms finalized and ready to go in the event of downtime, all preprinted clinical documentation forms must follow regulatory guidelines. Therefore, they need to be incorporated into any guideline and regulatory updates applied to the EHR.

Addressing order workflow is another priority during downtime. Physicians have become somewhat dependent on order sets to improve quality and efficiency in the ordering process. These order sets should be printed for ordering during downtime, or at the very least, as information resources. These should be maintained as close as possible to the electronic order set, as studies have shown that even the order of a pick list of items or the location of an order within an order set influences which ones are chosen.

As hectic and agonizing as the downtime episode may be, the recovery can be even worse. In addition to providing continual care for patients, the staff is burdened with the task of data reentry. In addition to improving workflow for clinicians during downtime, documentation tools that closely resemble the EHR will also facilitate data reentry and recovery. Items that can be reentered into the EHR can include, but are not limited to, paper clinical documentation, flow sheets (vitals, nursing assessments), orders, and problem lists. Thus, it is worthwhile to define a minimum data set that can be initially reentered into the system quickly so that other areas may begin data reentry. A second pass can then be taken to update remaining information. So, the practice needs to have a clear resource strategy that addresses what information will be entered into the EHR.

Depending on the time frame of the downtime episode, a substantial amount of information can be documented. Subject to the features of the EHR, it may be possible to input data normally entered discretely in a nondiscrete format. Some EHRs allow for storage and retrieval of scanned images. As such it may be possible for your group to scan large quantities of information and reference this information in the patient's EHR chart, and thus not add the burden of manually entering the information into the EHR. However, some critical information should be discretely entered back into the EHR. Examples include allergies or adverse drug reactions identified during the system downtime, problem list changes, and medication changes. Information that could affect coding and billing might also be important to reenter to aid in chart processing.

In an ideal world, development of an EHR is designed with downtime issues in mind. The tools developed within the EHR to improve and enhance quality and efficiency need to be addressed when designing downtime workflows and documents. Without an adequate downtime procedure in place and practice with these procedures, a downtime episode will adversely affect patient care.

 Lessons Learned

- Once a health system has a fully implemented EHR, care cannot continue "as usual" if the EHR goes down.
- Different stages of system outages should create clinical and operational triggers.
- Communication is essential in managing downtime.
- Health systems must prepare and practice for downtime.
- Downtime directly affects and is noticed by patients.

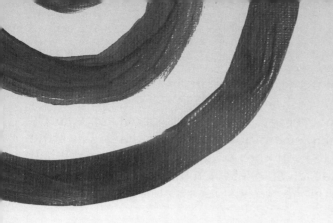

Weekends Are Not Just for Relaxing: Reconciliation after EHR Downtime

Editor: Justin Graham

Key Words:	Project Categories:	Lessons Learned Categories:
ambulatory, communication, downtime, EHR, training	ambulatory electronic health record (EHR)	communication, staffing resources, training

 ## Case Study

Interconnected Health Care is a large integrated delivery network that owns two larger (greater than 400 bed) hospitals, multiple smaller rural and community hospitals, and over 60 clinics. A "big-bang" implementation was its strategy for an electronic health record (EHR) implementation, with all functionality rolled out to all clinical staff at each location on the same day. The go-live schedule was designed to implement a group of clinics first, and then the hospital to which those clinics primarily referred.

The system had only been implemented in two 60-bed rural hospitals, including their clinics, plus several clinics associated with a larger community hospital when the first unscheduled downtime occurred. It lasted for several hours on a Sunday afternoon, when none of the ambulatory sites were open.

If an end-user had been working in the system when it went down, they had no idea there was anything wrong, but the moment they secured their workstation or ended their session they could not get back in. The call went out immediately to the hospitals to log out and implement downtime procedures. Once the system came back online, it rebooted with the backup from the moment it had gone down. Leadership breathed a sigh of relief when the system was back up and focused their recovery efforts on the two hospitals that had been affected. That is until Monday morning.

Providers in every live clinic came into work on Monday morning and found many of their completed charts still open. Multiple providers called the help desk with complaints that they had finished the charts over the weekend and their work had been lost. The information about the downtime eventually reached the clinics' leadership, who then had to pass on the information that any data entered during the downtime had been lost. Since the clinics were closed at the time the downtime occurred, no one had reached out to any of the ambulatory staff. The estimate of charts with lost data numbered in the hundreds, and the providers were extremely unhappy about not just the lost data, but also the amount of effort that had to be duplicated to reenter the information. Some clinics offered to have other staff perform the data entry, but most providers declined because they either had to enter subjective information or felt like it took so long to fill out the downtime forms that it would be easier and less risky to enter the information themselves the first time.

The negative word of mouth generated by the affected providers was perpetuated throughout the physician community at meetings for months. Leadership calculated this error in communication led to hundreds of hours of lost physician productivity and an inestimable loss of credibility and faith in the project and the system.

 ## Author's Analysis

Ensure that your communication plan for issues and emergencies includes all locations. This problem would likely have been prevented if the clinics' leadership had been notified and instructed to contact their providers about the downtime. A new business continuity plan was put into place with a set of downtime procedures that included clinic managers and physician leads as well as processes for downstream communication to all end-users via message alerts and pop-ups.

Do not underestimate the amount of time spent outside office hours performing work. The leadership assumed that because the number of open charts was small, their success with meeting the goal of charts being closed within 72 hours meant the providers were proficient with the system. This event highlighted the error in that assumption. The organization's Physician Engagement Team developed an Optimization Program after this event, with one goal being that of increasing provider efficiency and reducing the amount of time providers spent on their charting outside of office hours. This attempted to ameliorate some of the negative aftereffects of the event by reassuring physicians that organizational leadership cared about their work–life balance and wanted them to be able to finish their work in the same amount of time they did prior to the implementation of the new system.

 Editor's Commentary

Many advantages exist for using electronic medical records, but one disadvantage that was not foreseen by this hospital administration was the increased amount of time needed to document a case by physicians in the outpatient setting. In this situation, the physicians were not able to complete their charts in the normal time frame of the workweek, and thus were pushed to off-hour times, including the weekends, where this downtime event occurred. A lack of specific downtime procedures, specifically in the area of communication, resulted in an event that, while it had negligible effect on outpatient care, caused a significant issue with the outpatient providers.

Downtime can happen at any time and every system experiences some sort of downtime, crash, and other issues from time to time. It is how the downtime is planned for and handled that is important. Communication is vital to keep system users up to date about system downtime. A focus on best practices and guidelines to provide uninterrupted service in an efficient manner before, during, and after downtime is essential.

Communication channels are key, but they tend to be one-way and unsatisfactory for users. There are several fundamental aspects to consider when communicating during downtime:

- All stakeholders need to be involved in the development of downtime guidelines and procedures; they must be notified of any downtime, whether or not they are considered directly involved in the downtime.

- State clearly what the underlying cause of the downtime is (hardware, software, network, and such).

- Highlight likely consequences or lack thereof for the downtime (data loss, database corruption, prolonged downtime).

- Keep the tone very neutral. Do not place blame. Ideally this conveys acknowledgement of the problem with professionalism in addressing the issues leading to the downtime.

- If you send the announcement out by e-mail, your notification will be forwarded to several people. Make sure that the IT team and help desk understand the issues and consequences of the downtime. An executive summary to the C-suite helps them deal with any questions that can come their way. Technical details should be focused on those that understand them.

- Provide contact details (preferably someone who has the time in the midst of the downtime) for further questions, and ask for patience in the same sentence (this often works).

- Promise updates when the situation changes.

When the cause of the downtime has been addressed, send a summary including a list of all the possible consequences so that the users can review their data. This should also include the actions taken and changes implemented in the short term and those planned for the future ("lessons learned"), based on technical root cause analysis.

Training for downtime is vital. The first downtime training should occur when the system is being implemented. All system users should receive refresher training on a regular basis. Often overlooked, new employees hired after system implementation need to be trained on these procedures as part of their system training as well. In addition to all system users receiving regular training on downtime procedures, the channels of communication need to be tested on a regular basis to ensure they are viable options. E-mail addresses, phone extensions, personnel responsibilities, and physical office space can and frequently do change.

Once a downtime situation has been identified, consistent communication is vital throughout the downtime and its recovery among all stakeholders affected by the downtime. Regular testing and updating the communication channels is an absolute necessity to ensure that the system users adhere to all planned downtime procedures. Without key channels of communication, a well-planned downtime procedure will most like fail.

 Lessons Learned

- Ensure that communication plans for issues and emergencies includes all locations.
- Remember that work is often performed outside of office hours.
- Train for downtime.

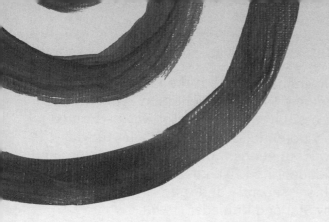

CHAPTER
30

104 Synergistic Problems: An Enterprise EHR

Editor: Eric Rose

Key Words:
electronic health record (EHR), downtime, end-user involvement, sociotechnical issues, vendor contracts, workflow

Project Categories:
ambulatory electronic health record (EHR), inpatient electronic health record (EHR)

Lessons Learned Categories:
contracts, leadership/governance, project management, technology problems, workflow

 ## Case Study

This HIT story describes an implementation of an integrated EHR system in a large university teaching hospital. The project started in 2001 and the implementation progressed slowly from one hospital unit to the next. The main parts of the system were Orfeus, for controlling and administrating healthcare processes and Medeia, for recording the care planning, realization, follow-up, and evaluation. The software provider had missed delivery dates and the parts delivered had not always met the original specifications. These challenges, combined with technical and integration problems, caused resistance among the hospital staff.

The resistance peaked in the surgical outpatient clinic and surgical inpatient unit where our story took place. The implementation was carried out in two of the surgical units during November 2005, but the situation was soon called a crisis by the staff members and the implementation came to a halt. In order to restart the project successfully, an assessment was performed to identify problems and recommend potential solutions. When studying the situation's problems, we interviewed surgeons, nurses, administration, and other EHR project stakeholders and identified 104 different issues of concern. These issues were classified into first-, second-, and third-order groups after the issue order model presented by Star and Ruhleder (1996).

First-Order Issues

First-order issues are often easily visible and solutions to them are practical. These issues were grouped according to the themes of redistribution of work resources and working time, arranging user training, and technical problems during the implementation.

After the implementation of the EHR, a main issue in information access was caused by workflows that were impeded. The process to use the EHR was slower than using the paper records at hand. One of the system features that slowed workflow was the structured character of the EHR. For example, there were more than 50 headings for recording a nursing action. One of the nurses described the situation as follows:

> Now I have to open Medeia, to open the nursing records. Now I'll create the record, that takes many clicks—like surgeons' names, date, and cause this and cause that. Then I'll have to choose the right headings, and then I can go and record the day visit by the patient ... and then I'll have to choose the next suitable heading... I have many workflow steps here, steps that I have never done before ... Before I just wrote, for example, 'covering letter' and 'breast cancer' on the paper and that was it.

The slowness of use affected workflows in various ways. For example, in the surgical outpatient department with continuous patient visits, half of the working time consisted of documenting patient records. In contrast, this took only about one-eighth of the working time in the surgical inpatient unit.

Second-Order Issues

Second-order issues can be caused by unpredictable contextual effects; that is, a collision or combination of two or more first-order issues. The unexpected effects may be caused by technical choices made or by the differences between the various cultures of practice that are working together in the implementation.

Combined effects of technical features that caused user resistance were, for example, the way the EHR logged off users, how the technical devices were arranged in the inpatient areas, or other problems that might have been caused by a constant need to repeatedly log in to the system. Constant technical problems caused the staff to think that the EHR did not ease their documenting load but rather interfered with their workflow and caused unwanted periods of waiting for the system to open or to find the next patient's data. Technical problems were further illustrated by the varied practices during downtime of the EHR system. During downtime, the patient records could be written as separate text files that could then be added into the EHR when the system was up again. Problems emerged when the separate text files were attached only as printouts to the paper version of the patient records and not entered into the EHR. The result was that the EHR was not necessarily up to date, and the staff could not trust the information in the EHR as complete or accurate.

Third-Order Issues

Third-order issues are often political or social by nature. Their nature dictates that these problems are also hard to solve. Such problems can be caused by the historical reasons behind the choices made in the implementation project or distinct features in the organizational culture.

The staff in the surgical clinic thought that they had no influence in system design and development. While working bedside, both a surgeon and a nurse might record information quite fluently and not consider whose user account was used to access the system. Problems of responsibility emerged when mistakes were made in the records. The one whose username was logged into the system was held responsible. On the other hand, surgeons feared that the slowness of use could cause malpractice in situations when patient information could not be accessed as easily as needed. A surgeon might have to make a decision on patient care with insufficient information.

 Author's Analysis

This conflicting situation was caused by a combination of multiple and intertwined sociotechnical issues. Emergence of such issues demanded attention on several levels in the organization, in this case, for example, by the information management department and hospital administration. The preliminary results suggest that social structures affecting the interaction in a hospital unit affect how the emergence of intertwined problems, handling the issues, and resolving the crisis takes place.

With previous manual patient records, the staff members were used to interpreting the paper records. Now with the EHR, feelings of insecurity emerged as well as the fear of ignorance as the previously usable interpretive schemes were insufficient in the changing context of interpretation. With the EHR, the patient information was "hidden" behind different headings of new nursing classifications and behind the views in the new system environment. Furthermore, the EHR was designed as independent system components. These components can work quite well by themselves, but the integration had caused some unexpected effects. Uncertainty combined with technical problems caused user resistance to reach its peak, and thus the implementation and use of the EHR came to a halt.

The case study shows that a new, unfamiliar information system can be accused of shortcomings or problems that may not actually be caused by the technology. In a crisis situation it is a human reaction to find a "scapegoat" that can be accused. Instead of simply labeling the new information system as a "scapegoat," we want to ask whether the implementation of an information system is a catalyst that makes it possible for other sociotechnical issues to emerge in the organizational context. The case study indicates that technical problems, such as slowness of use, can cause user resistance or at least increase users' doubt about the new information system. On the other hand, issues concerning professional values, such as fear of malpractice because of missing or inaccessible patient information, can lead to the decision not to use the system at all.

 ## Editor's Commentary

This fascinating case history of a HIT project that went seriously awry offers a smorgasbord of cautionary points. As the title suggests, it seems that every possible mishap that can occur in such a project took place.

It would be interesting to know what the decision-making process was for selecting the system used and its configuration. It seems likely, given the outcome, that involvement of the end-users—at least from the surgery department—was minimal. If there had been such end-user involvement, the usability issues described herein would likely have been recognized even before the purchasing decision was made, and the system would probably have been tailored to more closely match the true needs of the clinical staff.

The references to "slipped schedules" and the vendor-supplied software "not always meeting specifications" points to the importance of careful negotiation of vendor contracts. Such happenstances are not uncommon, and often are unavoidable (to be fair to the vendors), and this serves to underscore that organizations relying on vendor-supplied software should ensure that purchasing contracts clearly stipulate what remedies will be offered in such circumstances, and also include contingencies in their implementation plan for them.

The "issue order model" used to group the problems encountered in this project helps to differentiate problems that are straightforward and practical (though not necessarily easily solved) from those that involve interactions among several factors, such as the issue with adding the text files, which were created during periods of downtime, back to the EHR. This latter issue requires a consistent workflow outside the use of the EHR, which is often hard to achieve. The "third-order" issues in this case history describe a collision between the EHR system's characteristics and the professional realities of medical practice and serve to remind us of the high stakes where the safety of real patients, and the professional standing of real healthcare practitioners, are involved.

 ## Lessons Learned

- Stakeholder involvement in project planning and technology selection is critical.

- Technology-driven workflows must fit the needs of clinicians.

- Costs of project delays to both health systems and vendors should be reviewed prior to a technology implementation.

- HIT initiatives exist within the complex sociopolitical culture of the healthcare delivery system and are influenced positively and negatively by the organizations involved.

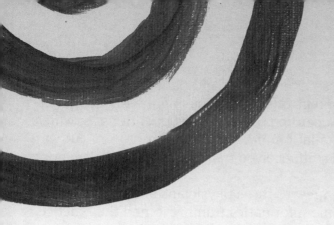

CHAPTER 31

"Meaningful Use"? A Small Practice EHR

Editors: Larry Ozeran and Jonathan Leviss

Key Words:
charge capture, decision support, efficiency, electronic health record (EHR), meaningful use, quality improvement, solo practice, training

Project Categories:
ambulatory electronic health record (EHR)

Lessons Learned Categories:
system design, technology problems, training

 Case Study

A young primary care physician, after practicing for several years at the same urban community health center where he had undergone residency training, decided it was time for a change. Despite having no experience in either solo private practice or in the use of EHR systems, he decided to establish his own solo practice and to use an EHR system from the first day, with no paper records. The decision to purchase and install an EHR system required a substantial capital investment and was a highly unusual step for a solo, private-practice physician in that city (itself a rare breed there).

The physician cited two main factors in the decision to adopt an EHR: efficiency and effective charge capture. "I wanted to be able to get my [visit] notes done quickly and bill electronically, and also not have the overhead for storage of paper charts." He also cited quality and patient-safety benefits such as drug-drug interaction warnings offered when using the EHR to generate prescriptions, and reminders regarding preventive interventions for which the patient is due. The initial installation and configuration of the EHR was uneventful, and the physician and staff received training from the EHR vendor at the time of initial installation.

Over several years, the practice grew to three physicians and two mid-level practitioners. A physician with some informatics training joined the practice. The new physician made some noteworthy observations:

- Although newer versions of the EHR system were available, the practice continued to use the version that was current when the practice was founded years before.

- Some processes (such as generating outside referrals) were being handled with paper, despite the capability of the EHR to handle them electronically.

- Certain configurable content, such as the rules on which automated reminders regarding preventive care are based, had not been changed since being automatically set during the initial software installation, despite changes in the evidence-based standards of care on which they were based.

- Certain basic security practices—such as assigning each user a separate user account and not sharing passwords—were not being followed.

- Many of the features of the software, some among them frequently cited as conferring the most important benefits of an EHR, were being used rarely or not at all: e-prescribing and computerized provider order entry (CPOE), assignment of discrete codes to patient diagnoses and problems, population-based reporting tools, creation of custom data fields to record discrete data of interest, and customization of documentation templates.

When these observations were pointed out to the practice's founding physician, he thought that although true, these observations were not of serious concern. "The program is effective for what I need it to do. I realize it can do a lot more, but I'm pretty happy with what I get out of it now, and I don't really have the time to get into all the details" of utilizing features such as those just mentioned. However, he acknowledged the potential value of such functionality, particularly in promoting patient safety and improving quality:

> I realize that a lot of the quality experts want us to use EHRs to do patient recalls, population-based care, and quality measurement … and I want to do all that too. I think sometimes what the experts don't realize is that physicians, particularly

those in private practice, where we're responsible for everything, need help just getting through the day taking care of our patients, and we focus on the aspects of an EHR that let us do that. I hope we can get to the rest of it someday soon.

Recently, the practice started taking steps to get more out of their EHR. They have upgraded to the latest version, started using the EHR's electronic prescribing capability (that is, electronic transmission of prescriptions directly to pharmacies, rather than printing or faxing prescriptions from the EHR), and are planning on participating in a quality improvement initiative that will provide reports on key quality measures extracted from data in their EHR. The growth of the practice to its current five providers has increased the level of product knowledge among the providers, as each gradually (often accidentally) discovers new aspects of how the EHR can be used and shares it with the others.

 ## Authors' Analysis

The case history raises the question of what "failure" means in the adoption and use of HIT. Specifically, this case illustrates that there are gradations of failure short of complete abandonment or deinstallation of a system, and that failure is, in some cases, a matter of context or expectations. The practice's founding physician absolutely does not see the practice's use of an EHR as a "failure." Quite to the contrary, the specific goals in mind when the decision to use an EHR was made, to allow documenting care more quickly than on paper without the expense of a transcriptionist, to avoid the space and associated expenses entailed by paper records, and to minimize accounts receivable through electronic claims submission, by any analysis were met.

On the other hand, many "experts" in clinical informatics and clinical quality improvement, blanching at the thought of the most valuable (from their perspective) features of an EHR going underused or unused, would look on this case history as a failure to obtain the maximum benefit from an EHR (Zhou et al. 2009). There are few published data on the frequency with which specific features of ambulatory EHRs are actually utilized (Simon et al. 2009). However, abundant anecdotal experience suggests that the case study is not unusual, and this might explain recently published data suggesting that use of an EHR alone is not associated with quality of care.

Practicing physicians and the experts do agree on one thing: the quality benefits obtained through capture and storage of discrete data in the EHR and leveraging of that data for just-in-time decision support and population-level care management are significant and worth striving toward. The question of "failure" in this case, then, becomes a simple matter of perspective on the pace of this evolution of the healthcare process. However, challenging questions remain: How can EHRs be engineered so that these more "advanced" features are easier to use? How can the organization of healthcare services and their financing be restructured to increase the feasibility of more effective utilization of EHR technology? How can physicians, particularly busy ones trying to run a practice on their own and who may need training and assistance, be identified, and how can that training and assistance be provided to them?

 ## Editor's Commentary

The author's final questions are particularly important since the passage of the American Recovery and Reinvestment Act of 2009 (ARRA). Under ARRA, the US federal government committed approximately $20 billion to HIT initiatives, including billions for payment incentives for physicians to use EHRs in a manner that provides "meaningful use." As this book goes to print, the exact definition of, or requirements for, "meaningful use" are being debated by every US healthcare, healthcare technology, and healthcare informatics organization; the US Office of the National Coordinator for Health IT (ONC), under the Department of Health and Human Services, will ultimately clarify the definition of "meaningful use," and, in effect, add commentary to cases such as the one described herein.

Regarding the assessment of this case study, it might be instructive to know how much the physician paid for the system and support services as a percentage of revenues. Similarly, it might be useful to know how many patients the physician was seeing and how many hours were spent in the clinic each day compared to after being in solo practice for one year. This would provide more concrete evidence that the system was, in fact, a success for the goals the physician initially set.

The bigger issue, as the author has accurately noted, is how this scenario plays out across the country, which has implications for our entire nation's healthcare system. As physicians and informaticists, we usually have two primary goals for EHRs: better care and lower costs. If we can provide the best care at the right time, we can likely achieve our goals. If decision support relies on old data or is not considered, both the nation's healthcare system and the patient lose. Unfortunately, all EHRs require training, and training requires time and resources. Most physicians currently feel overwhelmed by the amount of clinical and administrative work they must complete and often feel underpaid for their efforts. This is not a situation that encourages individuals to dedicate time without compensation to benefit the nation's health system, even if a quality of care "moral imperative" advocates such efforts. The next few years will demonstrate whether ARRA affects this pattern and whether "meaningful use" was attained by this practice or even is attainable by small physician practices in the United States.

 Lessons Learned

- A successful EHR meets the needs of the practice.
- EHR functionality may go unused or underutilized if the cost to implement appears to be greater than the benefit.
- Training requires a time commitment that must be seen as worthwhile to the trainee.
- EHR features that may benefit the healthcare system in aggregate may not be a priority for busy physicians who do not see the benefit as worth the cost.
- Increasing use of underused EHR features may require an easier user interface, repair of our healthcare system, or direct compensation to physicians for use.

Part III
Community Focus

"It's the Workflow, Stupid"

If you do not study your workflow ahead of time you will not be prepared for the disruptive changes CPOE causes. By hospital policy, when a patient went to the operating room, all preoperative orders were to be cancelled. Before CPOE, the ward clerk moved all active order sheets and the medication administration record to the back of the chart, safely out of the way and effectively discontinued. After the CPOE go-live, many postoperative patients had duplicate orders. Providers entered new postoperative orders, but no one had discontinued the existing preoperative orders. Without detection, order management workflow had shifted from the ward clerk to the provider, causing critical patient safety risks.

(Leviss 2008)

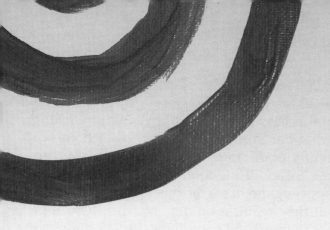

Push vs. Pull: Sharing Information across a Physician Referral Network

Editor: Jonathan Leviss

Key Words:	Project Categories:	Lessons Learned Categories:
communication, governance, provider portal, referring physician, tertiary care center	inpatient electronic health record (EHR), community-facing technologies	implementation approaches, system design, workflow

 Case Study

Over five years, a large multihospital integrated delivery healthcare system, with tertiary care centers of excellence, implemented an inpatient electronic health record (EHR) and a large medical archive repository. The organization had a large, experienced IT department, including development teams. Both the clinical teams and the IT department were very capable users and demonstrated the ability to create and support a variety of complex applications. Because of this, the quantity of electronic data and documents about each patient treated at the health system was considerable.

The health system relied on patient referrals for both inpatient volume and to maintain the organization's ability to support the tertiary care referral center. There were approximately 4,000 referring physicians and most of them did not have medical staff privileges at the health system hospitals. The health system provided easy referral access to care, but referring physicians were vocal and consistent about what became known as the "black hole," or their feeling that they were frequently uninformed about the care given to their patients at the referral center. In addition, communication about the handoff back to the community physician and expectations for follow-up care were largely missing. It was not that the organization did not have the will or understand the benefit associated with improved communication. Rather, the organization determined that finding solutions to improve communication was very difficult. Even with focused initiatives, such as capturing the primary care provider (PCP) at the time of admission, operations fell short, as evidenced by data indicating that staff recorded the PCP of the patient only about 60 percent of the time.

The organization spent some time deciding how to address this issue of information flow back to the referring physician population. There were discussions involving the use of the current EHR vendor's physician portal and another methodology that required more effort and a heavier reliance on data quality. The second option was a clinical messaging strategy, but it required a significant amount of continued development effort. The two solutions had fundamentally different methods to accomplish the task of provider communications. The physician portal was primarily a "come and get it" philosophy, making documents and results available to those who wanted to look for them (the pull method). The clinical messaging strategy focused on delivery of certain documentation to the physician (the push method). In the end, due to the difference in the time required to deploy each solution, the ease of deployment, and the cost, the final decision was to brand the available physician portal and roll that out as a strategy to combat the "black hole" phenomena.

The goals of the physician portal were to (1) improve communication of patient-care related information to referring physicians, (2) facilitate patient care and follow-up with the PCP after discharge, and (3) increase the accuracy of the recorded patient-physician relationship (that is, identify the PCP). To use the physician portal, providers were required to either be a member of the medical staff or remain referring providers and enter into an agreement that involved privacy, security, and use criteria. Once these requirements were met, the referring physician would be given a username and password for access. There was no classroom training available, but there were written training materials and an outreach liaison that could respond to questions, but did not have the capability to provide significant support. The password would reset every 90 days, due to system policy. Additionally, the physician portal permitted access to all patients and required a valid moral compass on the part of the provider to comply with the requirement that only patients that they were actively caring for would be viewed.

Although referring providers vocalized a need for improved follow-up information, further evaluation of their baseline experience (without the portal) was actually better than what was provided to them through the physician portal. Referring providers received copies of dictated discharge summaries, letters, and operative reports that were placed in an envelope and mailed to them. Within their offices, there was already a workflow process in which office staff would receive and triage the inbound information, marry it with the paper chart, and place the information in the same place every time. When it was convenient for the physician, they could locate new information, review historical information from their records (if necessary), write a quick note in the chart, and use sticky notes to notify staff of any actions that needed to be taken with the new information. This workflow process repeated itself several times a day and seamlessly integrated inbound documents from multiple locations (radiology, outpatient lab, telephone calls) into a single workflow for the physician. This was efficient, reproducible from day to day, and actually fulfilled the criteria for unified messaging, in which multiple communication pathways came to the individual as a single pathway, although with the shortcomings of paper-based records.

Geographically, the location of these offices varied from rural to urban and the size varied from single practitioners to multispecialty groups. Due to the nature of the healthcare industry in this region, these physicians had options to admit their patients to multiple hospitals in their community and when tertiary care referral was necessary, they had a choice of referral centers, as well. At this time, most of the offices had electronic practice management systems, but less than 10 percent had any EHR functionality.

The demographics, local and regional choices, and practice patterns resulted in a highly competitive environment where relationships with providers were extremely important. The physician portal was meant to enhance this relationship by providing the referring physicians with faster, greater, and more flexible access to follow-up information on their patients. Although anticipated to be a big success for this health system, actual results were quite different from the expectation.

Far fewer physicians even registered for access than expected because they just did not want to have to deal with another username and password. Of the physicians who did sign up, many of them did not attempt to access the portal and most of the remaining only tried once or twice. Since they were not using the portal every day, just remembering the URL to access the site became a frustrating chore for most, and the health system lost users when their passwords expired. Not knowing one's password meant calling a help desk at a number that was not easy to find. This was just too much hassle to locate a document on a patient that previously was found in the office chart. In addition, referring physicians felt they were doing extra work for information that the health system should be supplying to them (and in fact, used to deliver to them) rather than just providing a portal to look it up.

Even when the username and password issues were improved and some physicians frequently viewed documents, the feedback revealed another critical flaw in the deployment. A large part of the rationale for the physician portal was that it would make it easier for the health system's medical records department and might reduce some expenses. The health system could eliminate personnel stuffing envelopes, save on postage, and have more records available than before, but the physician practices had to absorb a newly fragmented workflow.

Reports still came to physician offices from many sources by fax, mail, and courier, requiring the continuation of the prior paper workflow. Now, the health system was also asking for a separate workflow for its portal-based documents. In order to integrate reports from the health system's portal into a patient's chart, the referring physician needed to search the portal for a new document, print out the document, and hand it to office staff to marry it with the paper chart. Next, the office staff would bring the full chart containing the printed document from the portal back to the physician for review. Alarmingly, this change alienated the physicians, made them less efficient, and actually impacted referrals. A frequently heard referring physician complaint was, "Why do I have to work so hard to find something that you should be delivering to me?"

Fortunately, in parallel to the early work with the physician portal, the health system continued to pursue the clinical messaging strategy. More evaluation of office workflow was done to understand how to deliver documentation electronically and seamlessly into the existing office workflow to minimize or extinguish disruption. This was accomplished with the clinical messaging system and enhanced by adding an additional layer of personal preferences that allowed the health system to leverage the customer relationship management (CRM) successes of other industries. For example, some physicians did not want to automatically receive operative notes, but discharge summaries were okay. Other physicians only wanted notification that their patients were in the Emergency Department (ED), but did not want to receive the ED note. What resulted was a very successful customer-focused deployment of messaging services that delivered documentation to physicians, only about their patients, the way they wanted to receive it. As more and more offices started to implement EHRs, work was planned on how to utilize the messaging infrastructure to insert documents directly into their EHRs. But there were customer service issues that needed to be solved before this could become widespread.

Author's Analysis

The health system failed to understand how users were thinking and did not initially monitor if what was deployed fit their needs. The customer-centric approach to design and deployment of technology is still in its infancy within healthcare, but this example demonstrated that it enhances adoption and is also a good business strategy. If you understand the needs and work environment of your users, you may find that you design, configure, and deploy your solutions differently than if you attempted to deploy a one-size-fits-all solution.

The workflow implications for the physician user population should have been understood before a particular solution was selected to solve the business problem. In this example, the business problem was fixing the "black hole." Portal access to documents could be a solution but there was not enough understanding of how it would be accessed and the environment it would be accessed from. It ended up having an opposite impact than what it was designed for. The health system should have focused more on the potential impact of the portal on referring providers and less on the personnel benefits from the deployment.

Insufficient effort and attention to data quality were committed to effectively personalize a service to a large group of care providers. Organizations must have a commitment to these operational components in order to make a more personalized deployment successful. But in at least this example of provider messaging, the organization's ultimate commitment to these operational details resulted in better physician relationships and increased referrals from those relationships.

If the health system had not assumed to know how the referral physicians were thinking or how they would respond to a certain situation or offering, but had asked, the project failure might have been averted.

Editor's Commentary

The author emphasizes the importance of tailoring a solution to the customer or end-user and asking the customer for input in solution design. Experiences in health IT repeatedly demonstrate that the complexity of our workflows and the high expectations of clinician users make buy-in and adoption of less than ideal solutions extremely challenging. Rather than simply asking the customer for input, engage the customer in the process. Health systems usually recognize that ED physicians must be involved in the planning, design, and go-live of ED rollouts; similarly, nurses must be part of project governance and implementation for medication systems. Community-based physicians, therefore, should be part of the project governance for community-facing initiatives. If members of the referral physician community had been involved in the project oversight, several key challenges might have been identified early in the project:

- Referring physicians likely would have known that they would still be managing paper documents even if the health system went "paperless."

- Referring physicians would have anticipated the concerns the hospital faced by requiring complex data access agreements for portal use.

- Referring physicians would have balked at the idea of requiring another password, especially one that changed frequently and was difficult to reset.

- The health system could have identified and addressed project barriers before wasting extensive resources and antagonizing the physician referral base.

Committees that identify barriers to a project early create the opportunity to address these barriers, compromise on solving them, not solve them, or even agree not to move forward on a project.

Without end-user adoption, projects with new technologies will never move forward. Sometimes the end-users are correct in rejecting the new technologies, but rarely is a health system correct in rejecting the input from the end-users.

 Lessons Learned

- Engage the customer before, during, and after deploying a new solution.

- Understand how customers are thinking and then closely monitor if deployed solutions fit their needs.

- Fully assess the workflow implications of a proposed solution prior to rollout.

- Ongoing effort and strict attention to detail is required to personalize service to a large group of care providers.

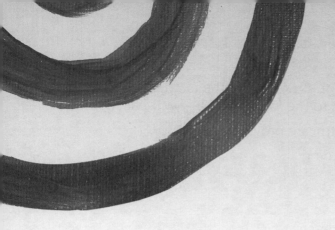

Loss Aversion: Adolescent Confidentiality and Pediatric PHR Access

Editor: Eric Poon

Key Words:	Project Categories:	Lessons Learned Categories:
confidentiality, chronic health conditions, pediatrics, PHR, privacy	community-facing technologies	communication, implementation approaches, system design

 Case Study

A large, nonprofit, multispecialist physician practice provides care for over 500,000 individuals in rural and urban communities spread over several states. Healthcare is provided at one acute care hospital and 25 primary care practices that encompass family medicine, pediatrics, and most medical and surgical subspecialists. Primary care is provided by nurse practitioners and family medicine physicians at all 25 clinics while pediatrics and subspecialty care are provided at seven clinics distributed over the service area.

The practice prides itself on being an early adopter of a clinical information system that includes an integrated personal health record (PHR). Extensive advertising is done that highlights the practice's use of health information technology (HIT) and how use of PHRs strengthens the patient–provider relationship. Patients have access to the following via a web-based portal:

- Secure messaging with healthcare providers
- Online appointment scheduling
- Laboratory and test results
- Immunization status
- Health maintenance reminders
- Problem lists, including drug allergies
- Postvisit summaries

In order to demonstrate its commitment to using PHRs, the practice provides financial incentives for providers who use secure messaging with patients. The practice also promotes the benefits of PHR use via posters in clinic waiting areas, recorded voice mail messages, and inserts included in mail sent to covered and prospective patients. Patient use of PHRs has gradually increased and in general patients and providers report satisfaction with PHRs.

More recently the practice moved all patients into a patient-centered medical home model. This care model continues to focus on use of the PHR as a means for patients to act in partnership with care providers in coordinating care. The practice's PHR system is seen as central to optimizing care.

One group of patients is kept from full participation in their care management. Citing concerns regarding privacy and confidentiality, the practice removes access to PHRs for adolescents as well as their parents and caregivers. Practice managers made this decision based on legal requirements restricting access to an adolescent's medical information. Current system functions make it difficult to control access to information in PHRs and meet Health Insurance Portability and Accountability Act (HIPAA) requirements fully. This means that families who were utilizing the PHR to schedule appointments, communicate with providers, access laboratory and test results, check immunization status, and monitor routine screening requirements lost those capabilities when their child turned 13. At the time this decision was made it was felt that parents would have no problem moving back to "traditional" methods of communicating with pediatric providers. Thus, no plans to mitigate unintended consequences were made.

Parents of adolescents living with chronic health conditions reported significant roadblocks to obtaining care following loss of parental access. Immunization reminders cannot be sent without PHR access. Unless there is an appointment scheduled or a specific request made via telephone, there is no way for parents to quickly determine immunization status for school or sports activities. Customer service staff and pediatric clinic administrators reported receiving complaints from parents who had been using online appointment scheduling. Other services have been impacted as well. As one parent stated, "The only way I knew we were moved from a case management model to the patient-centered medical home was because the complex case management nurse stopped calling me."

At this point, the practice has determined that there is a need to provide parents/caregivers access to some components of their child's PHR. However, due to other "pressing" HIT projects, work on this is not expected to begin until the next fiscal cycle.

 ## Author's Analysis

Review of the situation revealed the need for parents or caregivers to have access to certain functions of their child's PHR while ensuring that other areas of the PHR remain secure. Key lessons learned include the following:

- Development of a PHR for use in pediatrics involves security concerns not typically faced when developing PHRs in care settings that do not include pediatrics.

- Parent or caregiver needs for communication and information sharing must be considered when building pediatric PHRs.

- There is a need to provide access to the PHR for parents or caregivers to utilize online scheduling, check immunization status, communicate with providers, and view reminders and alerts as needed.

- Pediatric PHRs are much more complex to build and maintain than PHRs used for adult populations. The need for multiple layers of security is one reason for this complexity.

- Thorough testing is vital to ensure that protected health information is not inadvertently viewed by individuals who do not have authorization to do so.

 ## Editor's Commentary

This case demonstrates an episode of "growing pains" in an otherwise successful implementation of PHRs to support patient-centered care. As the PHR (or any form of HIT) is used more broadly, issues and risks are bound to emerge. In this particular case, privacy concerns were raised on behalf of adolescent patients who might not want their parents (or legal guardians) to access their records through the PHR. Because the PHR lacked the necessary functionality and processes to allow adolescents and their parents (or legal guardians) to negotiate and control who could access their records online, all PHR functionality was taken away for the adolescent population.

It is all too easy for us to second-guess the decision made by the "practice managers" to remove PHR access for adolescent patients. Although the HIPAA legislation was passed more than a decade ago, the hodgepodge of federal and state laws and regulations continue to evolve. Legislators, regulators, privacy advocates, legal experts, healthcare administrators, health information management professionals, and health information system professionals are all challenged to shape, interpret, and implement privacy laws and regulations. It is quite understandable that a practice manager whose domain expertise is in neither privacy nor HIT might err on the side of caution to minimize risk exposure to the practice.

With the benefit of hindsight, however, it might be instructive to examine more closely the decision-making process. It is not clear from the case whether the appropriate stakeholders were consulted before the decision was made. For example, did the medical director help the practice manager anticipate the impact of withdrawing PHR access on the care model the practice was transitioning towards? Were informatics professionals on hand to help define alternative approaches to the problem? Was the larger HIT community consulted on how other healthcare systems have addressed this concern? Did legal counsel help quantify the degree of risk if adolescents continued to use the PHR? It is very possible that the same decision might have been made even if additional resources were brought to the decision-making table. However, one could have expected practice leaders to appreciate the consequences of this decision and to spend the appropriate amount of time on making this decision.

If we assume that no technical solution was immediately available within the PHR to address the privacy concerns, other process-driven approaches might have allowed the practice to preserve PHR access for adolescents and their parents (or legal guardians). For example, the practice staff could ask adolescent patients (while alone from their parents or legal guardians) whether they wanted continued access to their PHR. If the practice could develop simple decision aids (for example, a short list of benefits and risks for the adolescents, or talking points for staff), the resource draw on the practice might be minimal. Alternatively, PHR access could be taken away for all adolescent patients and be granted back only if both the adolescent and adult review the benefits and risks of PHR access. While these and other alternatives might not have mitigated all the risks, they may be sufficient as interim measures as technical solutions are developed.

We might infer that the practice was surprised by the negative reactions from patients and their parents (or legal guardians) when their PHR access was taken away. In retrospect, insights from the field of behavioral economics might have anticipated this as people have a tendency to strongly prefer avoiding losses to acquiring gains, a phenomenon known as "loss aversion." If PHR access had never been offered to the adolescent population, the patients and their parents (or legal guardians) might never have complained. However, when functionality is taken away, one could expect dissatisfaction from at least a vocal minority. Had the practice anticipated this, they could have pursued more aggressively mitigation strategies, such as communicating the loss of PHRs proactively to patients and their parents or guardians and reminding parents or legal guardians how they could otherwise obtain immunization records. Alternatively, a summary of the patient's record (such as medications and immunizations) could be proactively given to the patient at every visit.

 Lessons Learned

- PHR use in pediatrics involves unique privacy and confidentiality concerns.
- Parent or caregiver needs for communication and information sharing must be considered when building PHRs.
- Stakeholder input is critical for successful HIT initiatives.

Failure to Scale: A Teaching Module

Editor: Gail Keenan

Key Words:	Project Categories:	Lessons Learned Categories:
ambulatory electronic health record (EHR), documentation, medical education, student, testing, user interface	community-facing technologies, infrastructure and technology	technology problems

 Case Study

Students at our institution have read access to numerous clinical electronic record systems, but none of these specifically augment medical education. Students' electronic data-recording opportunities are almost nonexistent. For several years we have developed student patient record (SPR) programs that record a small amount of information about students' clinical encounters. These modest contents have provided educational decision support and summary statistics in primary care settings. We attempted to expand SPR use to all third-year clinical rotations.

SPR version 5 was a stable program built in Satellite Forms 5 and tailored to loaned Palm Tungsten C handheld devices. For new patients, students could

197

record demographics, then record diagnoses arranged by patient type, often using one tap per diagnosis, without scrolling or typing. Family Medicine's new patient types were distinguished by age: Adult, Teen, Child, Infant, and Baby. In SPR 5, students recorded 70 percent of ambulatory care diagnoses from new patient screens, and could find additional diagnoses in shallow tree structures or alphabetized lists. Students received small rewards for thorough, statistically plausible documentation.

We encountered a serious limitation in the design environment while expanding the number of screens representing diagnoses as check boxes in SPR 6: Satellite Forms 6 was recompiling the global script anew for every check box, causing extremely long compile times. We were forced to remove the reminder system from the global script while waiting for the Satellite Forms vendor to repair the problem in version 7. Every student was loaned a Tungsten E2 computer. These affordable handheld devices proved at least three times slower than the Tungsten C when opening SPR or filtering long lists.

We had no wireless network. Students sometimes compromised data gathering by changing key user identification, declining to install a critical update, or ignoring the program completely. We generally had to detect and react to these events in person.

Other clerkships wanted students to document completion of explicit goals rather than complete patients. Although much of the SPR 5 interface was faster than paper for recording diagnoses in primary care settings, and all goals were represented similarly in SPR 6, goals were not actually listed or tracked. Furthermore, students changed clinical settings approximately every four weeks, so they regularly had to learn new button arrangements tailored to new courses. Course directors voiced concerns that students were spending more time on documentation than seeing patients.

We had relied on infrared beaming and regular contact with small numbers of students to collect data from SPR 5. Several clerkships had intermittent contact with large groups of students using SPR 6. Infrared beaming was extremely cumbersome in these circumstances.

A web-based status report was the only verification that a student had met course goals. We had only 0.4 full-time equivalent staff (FTE) divided between two individuals to develop and maintain SPR 6, a server, and the reporting programs. Personal distractions delayed the delivery of the reporting system. When reports became available, some additional goal documentation and data collecting problems were exposed. Efforts to appease frustrated students included suspending SPR documentation and allowing them to purchase the Tungsten E2s at a discount.

SPR 7 attempted to address all SPR 6 problems with the exception of wireless networking. SPR 7 disposed of button arrays and added security, dynamic list management, goal tracking and goal-based documentation, decision support, dynamic input area support, and interactive help features. The SPR 7 interface was tailored to the fastest affordable and available Palm device, the TX, running the new nonvolatile file system and the Garnet 5.4.9 operating system (OS).

We sought speed enhancements using extensions to Satellite Forms 7. Late in testing we discovered situations causing SPR 7 to crash with a cache error on the TX. This seemed to occur when extensions encountered boundary conditions. Cache errors were malignant. After suffering one crash on a TX, SPR 7 crashed at progressively earlier steps, quickly becoming useless. One day before scheduled deployment we found more cache errors and could not correct these in the ensuing week. Our Palm-based project was canceled.

 Author's Analysis

We experienced numerous difficulties with SPR 6 and 7, nearly all related to scaling a previously successful project in a narrow domain to more courses, more simultaneous student users, and more administrators' needs. Some key points follow:

- Participants' goals need to be reconciled or managed proactively. Most of our institution was interested in goal tracking whereas we saw much more promise in demonstrating the benefits of more thorough, patient-oriented documentation. We are rebuilding SPR for Windows Mobile with our attention directed first to meeting the documentation needs of administrators. From the student perspective, deploying SPR 6 without the reminder system scuttled the last reason we could offer for thorough documentation.

- An interface that works when learned once may not work when users must relearn it often. If the interface content changes, it should provide some other consistency, such as alphabetized or structured lists. We emphasize that this lesson may not apply to practicing physicians. The diminutive SPR 5/6 interface is faster than paper for recording 70 percent of students' primary care diagnoses when they are graded on completeness. If a user consistently works in a domain having predictable clusters of recordable concepts, then similar interfaces may be optimal.

- Adequate resource allocations are essential. Wireless or Internet-based services are almost indispensable for deploying updates and collecting data from many users. Important projects require more developer depth and redundancy than we had.

- Early and aggressive testing on the target platform is invaluable. Hardware and operating system changes can interact badly with software tools. Although we waited more than one year from its first release to use the TX and Garnet 5.4.9, and thought that our development tools were stable on the new platform, we were wrong.

 ## Editor's Commentary

This story is an example of what many others have experienced when there is insufficient planning before the development of information technology (IT). Although the story does not describe the initial SPR development phase, it seems apparent that proper planning could have produced better outcomes. As the field of IT grows in healthcare, the importance of planning and sufficient testing cannot be overstated. Abandoning a technology that was not built to scale fuels increases in the already out-of-control healthcare costs with the corresponding adverse implications for patients, clinicians, and organizations.

Indeed, it is nearly impossible to isolate all of the hardware, software, user, content, and political factors that might influence how an application will be used across time. It is also outlandish to focus on meeting only the immediate needs of the user without attention to the reality that user needs naturally grow and change across time. Our team has managed to avoid early obsolescence with our IT innovations by keeping a 10-year development plan current. We carefully envision and create plans about what we want based on what we think is possible in 10 years, adjusting the plan each year. As we have found, creating a plan to sustain an IT innovation for a decade has forced us to create a flexible product that can readily handle multiple types of contingencies both known and unknown. Of course there will always be some costs associated with evolving a product over time; however, we believe vigilant and creative long-term planning are key to keeping overall costs to a minimum.

 ## Lessons Learned

- Considering the long-term possibilities of an IT innovation prior to development ensures the product can grow and scale with minimal costs, including changes in hardware, software, policies, users, and content.

- Adequate testing with all types of users under the conditions of use is essential for evaluating the true value of any IT innovation.

- Seeking input of users, although essential, is insufficient to build successful IT innovations.
- A solid ongoing collaborative partnership between technical and clinical experts is equally as important.
- Project planning should be an ongoing aspect of any HIT initiative, with governance document changes as necessary.

Part IV
Conclusion

The Interpersonal Stuff

When the button was pushed at EHR go-live everything suddenly changed—for just about everyone. The intense stress caused different people to react in different ways. Sometimes emotions ran high and people became angry, verbally attacking EHR leadership. Having a large supply of friends came in very handy; so did having patience and empathy. Frequently the vocal people had extremely important points underneath their rhetoric.

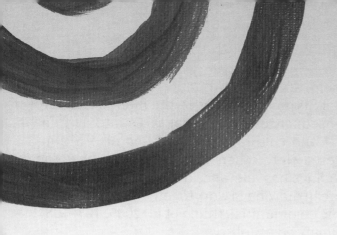

Theoretical Perspective: A Review of HIT Failure

S. Silverstein, B. Kaplan, J. Leviss, and L. Ozeran

Health information technology (HIT) projects are highly complex social endeavors in unforgiving medical environments that happen to involve computers, not IT projects that happen to involve clinicians. Knowledge about people, organizations, implementation, and maintenance issues has grown over the years, both within medical informatics itself and through contributions from other disciplines (Ash et al. 2008; Kaplan and Shaw 2004). There is an emerging consensus that problems are caused by social, cultural, and financial issues, and hence, are more managerial than technical (Kaplan and Harris-Salamone 2009).

In addition to the observed and reported stories of HIT failures within organizations, there is a theoretical framework that is both practical and well-grounded in research (Kaplan 2001a). From the many useful theories and frameworks (Kaplan and Shaw 2004), two are popular among informaticists analyzing the kinds of issues that our case studies illustrate. One is Rogers's Diffusion of Innovation (Rogers 2003) and its extensions to address gaps relevant to HIT implementations (Lorenzi et al. 2008). Another is sociotechnical theory (Harrison et al. 2007). Both are social interactionist theories (Kaplan 2001b). Social interactionist theories in informatics were developed and extended by the late Rob Kling, the father of social informatics (SI), during his tenure at the University of California, Irvine, and then at Indiana University.

Kling thought that many information and communications technology (ICT) professionals have an inadequate understanding of ICT, the actions and interactions of people who use them, and the organizational and social contexts in which they are used. Social informatics refers to the interdisciplinary study of the design, uses, and consequences of ICTs that takes into account their interaction with institutional and cultural realities. Kling also recommended that communicating SI research to others is important because the value of SI theory, insights, and findings has relevance across a range of disciplines. He defines a major challenge in drawing SI work together and beginning to make it known to other academic communities (Kling et al. 2005, 107–108).

The principles of SI can be summarized as follows:

- The context of ICT use directly affects its meaning and roles.
- ICTs are not "value neutral"—they create winners and losers.
- ICT use leads to multiple and often paradoxical effects that are multifarious and unpredictable.
- ICT use has ethical aspects.
- ICTs are configurable.
- ICTs follow trajectories, often favoring the status quo.
- ICTs coevolve before and after implementation; all are social activities.

Most important of all is critical thinking about ICT projects; that is, developing the ability to examine ICTs from perspectives that do not automatically and implicitly adopt the goals and beliefs of the groups that commission, design, or implement specific ICTs. Critical thinking also entails developing an ability to reflect on issues at a number of levels and from more than one perspective (Kling et al. 2000, 123). For these reasons, according to Marc Berg, one of sociotechnical theory's main expositors, the idea of "success factors" becomes problematic, as they entail the idea that a fixed list of activities and characteristics will ensure "success." "Success" depends both on the point of view of users who may differ in whether and to what degree they consider a system "successful," and on the specific situation and the complex processes of addressing the kinds of insights Kling identified (Berg 2001).

These principles explain why Kaplan's review of individual, organizational, and social issues identified the fit of information and communication technologies with other contextual issues surrounding their development, implementation, and use as crucial to their success. Research on these principles include the importance of fit in the following areas:

- Workflow and routines
- Clinicians' level of expertise
- Values and professional norms

- Institutional setting, history, and structure
- Communication patterns, organizational culture, status relationships, control relationships, division of labor, work roles, and professional responsibility
- Cognitive processes
- Congruence with existing organizational business models and strategic partners
- Compatibility with clinical patient encounter and consultation patterns
- The extent to which models embodied in a system are shared by its users

Authors have also addressed (in various ways) fit between information technology and how individuals define their work, user characteristics, and preferences (such as information needs), the clinical operating model under which a system is used, and the organization into which it is introduced. Others have focused on interrelationships among key components of an organization, (that is, organizational structure, strategy, management, people's skills, and technology) and compatibility of goals, professional values, needs, and cultures of different groups within an organization, including developers, clinicians, administrators, and patients. In addition, studies have been done on ways in which informatics applications embody values, norms, representations of work and work routines, assumptions about usability, information content and style of presentation, and links between medical knowledge and clinical practice, and how these assumptions influence system design (Kaplan and Shaw 2004; Kaplan 2001b).

Kaplan's research also identified the same four barriers—insufficient funding, technology, and knowledge; poor project management; the organization of medicine and healthcare; and physician resistance—blamed for lack of diffusion of ICT in healthcare since the 1950s. These barriers are characterized by looking to external causes for the problems in our field (Kaplan 1987). They are evidence of beliefs Kling and Iaconno characterized as computerization movements that too often characterize the driving forces behind HIT (Kling and Iaconno 1988). Among these beliefs is the technologically deterministic view that ICT in and of itself, not SI principles, will cause organizational and individual change in healthcare delivery and the practice of medicine. A close relative of technological determinism is the "magic bullet" theory, where people believe they are change agents if they initiate or develop IT because they think IT itself has the power to create organizational change. These people describe IT as a "magic bullet" and believe that they have built the gun (Markus and Benjamin 1997).

Unfamiliarity with the findings of SI research and beliefs in technologic determinism directly contribute to healthcare IT failure.

Some authors in the healthcare informatics sphere have begun to challenge the dominant paradigm (Koppel et al. 2005; Han et al. 2005), but not without raising significant controversy and receiving considerable criticism (despite significant problems in local and national EHR initiatives in the United States and abroad) (Freudenheim 2004; Peel and Rose 2009). Yet there is new interest in information on HIT difficulties, as illustrated by the success of the first edition of HIT *or Miss*, many presentations on HIT failure at small and large professional society meetings, inquiries by members of the US Congress into HIT failures (Conn 2010), and opinion articles in leading national newspapers and academic journals.

Assessments of failures must continue and the lessons learned must be shared broadly if we are to meet the call to leverage HIT to dramatically improve health systems across the United States and the world.

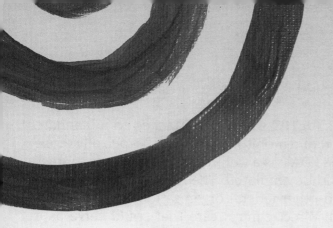

CHAPTER 36

Call to Action

How do we as an industry collectively get wisdom? State or federal regulators and accrediting organizations could require us to file reports about health information technology (HIT) failures, whether or not they involve patient safety events. Given the size of the federal investment in HIT through the American Recovery and Reinvestment Act (ARRA), often cited as the single largest investment in any national initiative, it is surprising that this oversight has not already been established. In 2010, AMIA published a position paper addressing the legal impediments and contractual gag laws health systems face when trying to openly report adverse events that involve HIT, especially when problems involve information technology design or configuration. AMIA's recommendations included a declaration that "patient safety should trump all other values" (Goodman 2011). Additionally, in the fall of 2011, the Institute of Medicine (IOM) issued a report on health IT and patient safety and called for the US Department of Health and Human Services to establish and fund a "Health IT Safety Council." The Council would catalogue and report adverse events as a result of HIT (IOM 2011).

As important as these approaches are to learning about the risks of HIT, we do not need to wait in order to learn from our own or each other's HIT failures. Each and every healthcare organization, from large hospital systems to small physician practices, each HIT service firm, and every HIT vendor has a responsibility to create a process that transparently identifies, tracks, and evaluates HIT failures and the adverse affects to patients and organizations. A first step involves internal monthly conferences to review projects that failed and to identify critical lessons for both current and future efforts. Participation should be broad, including all contributors to the project. Additionally, active efforts should be started to monitor existing projects for warning signs of failure and suggesting solutions before adverse outcomes occur. Hotlines could be created to alert management to projects, just as exist for safety monitoring in other aspects of healthcare.

Most importantly, federal funds for HIT should be attached to a mandate that healthcare organizations report and monitor HIT failures, especially those that directly affect patient care. The FDA has a well-developed process to track medication safety issues that could be emulated. The Agency for Healthcare Research and Quality (AHRQ) and other federal organizations support morbidity and mortality rounds about direct clinical care that could serve as a model for discussing HIT failures. The Office of the National Coordinator for Health Information Technology (ONC) or the Centers for Medicare and Medicaid Services (CMS) should mandate HIT failure reporting as a component of Meaningful Use attestation. The ARRA-funded Regional Extension Centers (RECs) could support a similar effort for small physician practices across the United States.

There are many ways to share lessons learned from HIT failures and the biggest failure would be to continue to repeat the known errors over and over again.

Appendices

Magical Thinking

Clinician: "I'd appreciate it if you'd arrange all my patients in my coverage list by hair color... What? You didn't include information about hair color as structured data in the EHR—ask the vendor for an enhancement; better yet—scan in a color picture, and use color sensors to populate the hair color. Then look up their home zip code and find all nearby hairdressers. Send an automatic e-mail requesting an appointment three days after discharge."

CMIO: "No problem".

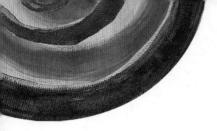

Appendix A

HIT Project Categories

Ambulatory Electronic Health Record (EHR)

- Chapter 22: All Automation Isn't Good
- Chapter 23: Clinician Adoption
- Chapter 24: Start Simple…Maybe
- Chapter 25: Leadership and Strategy
- Chapter 26: Designing Custom Software for Quality Reports
- Chapter 28: All Systems Down…What Now?
- Chapter 29: Weekends Are Not Just for Relaxing
- Chapter 30: 104 Synergistic Problems
- Chapter 31: "Meaningful Use"?

Inpatient Electronic Health Record (EHR)

- Chapter 1: Build It with Them, Make It Mandatory, and They Will Come
- Chapter 2: One Size Does Not Fit All
- Chapter 3: Hospital Objectives vs. Project Timelines
- Chapter 4: Clinical Quality Improvement or Administrative Oversight
- Chapter 5: Disruptive Workflow Disrupts the Rollout
- Chapter 6: Anatomy of a Preventable Mistake
- Chapter 7: Failure to Plan, Failure to Rollout
- Chapter 8: Basic Math
- Chapter 9: Technological Iatrogenesis from "Downtime"
- Chapter 10: Trained as Planned
- Chapter 12: Collaboration Is Essential

Community-Facing Technologies (Physician and Consumer)

Computerized Provider Order Entry (CPOE)

Electronic Medication Administration Record (eMAR)

- Chapter 3: Hospital Objectives vs. Project Timelines
- Chapter 5: Disruptive Workflow Disrupts the Rollout
- Chapter 6: Anatomy of a Preventable Mistake
- Chapter 7: Failure to Plan, Failure to Rollout
- Chapter 8: Basic Math
- Chapter 9: Technological Iatrogenesis from "Downtime"

Pharmacy IS

- Chapter 5: Disruptive Workflow Disrupts the Rollout
- Chapter 6: Anatomy of a Preventable Mistake
- Chapter 7: Failure to Plan, Failure to Rollout
- Chapter 8: Basic Math
- Chapter 9: Technological Iatrogenesis from "Downtime"

Infrastructure and Technology

- Chapter 11: Device Selection—No Other Phase Is More Important
- Chapter 16: A Single Point of Failure
- Chapter 17: Vendor and Customer
- Chapter 18: Ready for the Upgrade
- Chapter 34: Failure to Scale

Laboratory Information Systems

- Chapter 13: Lessons beyond Bar Coding
- Chapter 14: Sticker Shock
- Chapter 22: All Automation Isn't Good

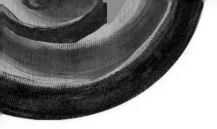

Appendix B

Lessons Learned Categories

Communication

Contracts

Data Model

Implementation Approaches

Leadership/Governance

System Configuration

System Design

Technology Problems

Training

- Chapter 2:   One Size Does Not Fit All
- Chapter 9:   Technological Iatrogenesis from "Downtime"
- Chapter 10:   Trained as Planned
- Chapter 13:   Lessons beyond Bar Coding
- Chapter 23:   Clinician Adoption
- Chapter 28:   All Systems Down…What Now?
- Chapter 29:   Weekends Are Not Just for Relaxing
- Chapter 31:   "Meaningful Use"?

Workflow

- Chapter 2:   One Size Does Not Fit All
- Chapter 4:   Clinical Quality Improvement or Administrative Oversight
- Chapter 5:   Disruptive Workflow Disrupts the Rollout
- Chapter 6:   Anatomy of a Preventable Mistake
- Chapter 7:   Failure to Plan, Failure to Rollout
- Chapter 11:   Device Selection—No Other Phase Is More Important
- Chapter 12:   Collaboration Is Essential
- Chapter 13:   Lessons beyond Bar Coding
- Chapter 14:   Sticker Shock
- Chapter 15:   If It Ain't Broke, Don't Fix It
- Chapter 22:   All Automation Isn't Good
- Chapter 23:   Clinician Adoption
- Chapter 27:   If It's Designed and Built by One, It Will Not Serve the Needs of Many
- Chapter 30:   104 Synergistic Problems
- Chapter 32:   Push vs. Pull

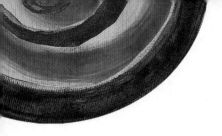

Appendix C

Text References and Bibliography of Additional Resources

References

Ash, J.S., N.R. Anderson, and P. Tarczy-Hornoch. 2008. People and organizational issues in research systems implementation. *Journal of the American Medical Informatics Association* 15(3):283–289.

Bakken, S. 2001. An informatics infrastructure is essential for evidence-based practice. *Journal of the American Medical Informatics Association.* 8:199–201.

Berg, M. 2001. Implementing information systems in health care organizations: myths and challenges. *International Journal of Medical Informatics.* 64:143–156.

Conn J. 2010. Grassley queries hospitals about IT vendors, 'gag order' contract clauses. Modern Healthcare. http://www.modernhealthcare.com/article/20100120/INFO/301209999/0#.

Freudenheim, M. 2004 (April 6). Many hospitals resist computerized patient care. *New York Times.*

Glaser, J. 2005 (June 13). Success factors for clinical information system implementation. *Hospital and Health Networks' Most Wired Magazine.*

Goodman, K.W., Berner, E.S., Dente, M.A., Kaplan, B., Koppel R., et al. 2011. Challenges in ethics, safety, best practices, and oversight regarding HIT vendors, their customers, and patients: a report of an AMIA special task force. *Journal of the American Medical Informatics Association* 18(1):77–81.

Han, Y.Y., J.A. Carcillo, S.T. Venkataraman, R.S.B. Clark, R.S. Watson, T.C. Nguyen, H. Bayir, and R.A. Orr. 2005. Unexpected increased mortality after implementation of a commercially sold computerized physician order entry system. *Pediatrics* 116:1506–1512.

Hann's On Software. 2008. Hann's On Software HL7 Interface Specification. Documentation Version: 4-1-2008.

Harrison, M.I., R. Koppel, S. Bar-Lev. 2007. Unintended consequences of information technologies in health care—an interactive sociotechnical analysis. *Journal of the American Medical Informatics Association* 14(5):542–549.

Institute for Safe Medication Practices. 2007. High-Alert Medication Feature: Anticoagulant safety takes center stage in 2007. ISMP *Medication Safety Alert!* http://www.ismp.org/newsletters/acutecare/articles/20070111.asp.

Institute of Medicine of the National Academies. 2011. *Health IT and Patient Safety: Building Safer Systems for Better Care*. Washington D.C.: The National Academies Press.

Kaplan, B. 1987. The medical computing 'lag': Perceptions of barriers to the application of computers to medicine. *International Journal of Technology Assessment in Health Care* 3(1):123–136.

Kaplan, B. 2001a. Evaluating informatics applications—Review of the clinical decision support systems evaluation literature. *International Journal of Medical Informatics* 64(1):15–37.

Kaplan, B. 2001b. Evaluating informatics applications—Social interactionism and call for methodological pluralism. *International Journal of Medical Informatics* 64(1):39–56.

Kaplan, B. and K.J. Harris-Salamone. 2009. Health IT project success and failure: Recommendations from literature and an AMIA workshop. *Journal of the American Medical Informatics Association* 16(3):291–299.

Kaplan, B. and N. Shaw. 2004. Future directions in evaluation research: People, organizational, and social issues. *Methods of Information in Medicine* 43(3–4): 215–231.

Keenan GM, E. Yakel, K. Dunn Lopez, D. Tschannen, and Y. Ford. 2012. Challenges to nurses' efforts of retrieving, documenting and communicating patient care. *Journal of the American Medical Informatics Association*. PMID: 22822042.

Kling, R., H. Crawford, H. Rosenbaum, S. Sawyer, S. Weisband. 2000. Learning from social informatics: information and communication technologies in human contexts. Center for Social Informatics, Indiana University. http://rkcsi. indiana.edu/archive/SI/Arts/SI_report_Aug_14.doc.

Kling R., H. Rosenbaum, and S. Sawyer. 2005. *Understanding and Communicating Social Informatics: A Framework for Studying and Teaching the Human Contexts of Information and Communication Technologies*. Medford, NJ: Information Today Press. 107–108.

Kling, R. and S. Iaconno. 1988. The mobilization of support for computerization: The role of computerization movements. *Social Problems* 34:226–243.

Koppel, R., J.P. Metlay, A. Cohen, B. Abaluck, A.R. Localio, S.E. Kimmel, B.L. Strom. 2005. Role of computerized physician order entry systems in facilitating medication errors. *Journal of the American Medical Association* 293: 1197–1203.

Leviss, J. and C. Cole. "Physician Leaders—Why the HIT struggle?" Presented at HIMSS Annual Conference. February 2008.

Lorenzi, N.M., L.L. Novak, J.B. Weiss, C.S. Gadd, and K.M. Unertl. 2008. Crossing the implementation chasm: A proposal for bold action. *Journal of the American Medical Informatics Association* 15(3):290–296.

Markus, M.L. and R.I. Benjamin. 1997. The magic bullet theory in IT-enabled transformation. *Sloan Management Review* 38(2):55–68.

Novak, J. 2012 (August 28). HIMSS Industry Solution Webinar: IT Projects Have a 70% Failure Rate: Don't Let Your Hospital IT Projects Fail. Chicago: HIMSS

Obama, B. Address to Joint Session of the Congress, February 24, 2009. Public Papers of the Presidents of the United States. Washington, D.C.: Government Printing Office, 2009. http://www.gpo.gov/fdsys/pkg/PPP-2009-book1/pdf/PPP-2009-book1-Doc-pg145-2.pdf.

Ong, K. 2011. *Medical Informatics—An Executive Primer*, 2nd ed. Chicago: HIMSS.

Peel, L. and D. Rose. 2009. MPs point to 'further delays and turmoil' for £12.4 billion NHS computer upgrade. Times Online. http://www.thetimes.co.uk/tto/news/uk/article1937417.ece.

Pizzi, R. 2007. EHR adoption an 'ugly process,' but CCHIT can improve appeal. *Healthcare IT News*. http://www.healthcareitnews.com/news/ehr-adoption-ugly-process-cchit-can-improve-appeal.

PRINCE2. 2013.What is PRINCE2? http://www.prince2.com/what-is-prince2.asp.

Rogers, E.M. 2003. *Diffusion of Innovations*, 5th ed. New York: The Free Press.

RTI Health, Social, and Economics Research. 2002. *The Economic Impacts of Inadequate Infrastructure for Software Testing Final Report*. Gaithersburg, MD: National Institute of Standards and Technology.

Saroyan, W. 1971. *The Human Comedy*. New York: Random House.

Silverstein, S. 2006. Access patterns to a website on healthcare IT failure. AMIA 2006 Annual Meeting, poster session.

Simon, S.R. C.S. Soran, R. Kaushal, C.A. Jenter, L.A. Volk, E. Burdick, P.D. Cleary, E.J. Orav, E.G. Poon, and D.W. Bates. 2009. Physicians' usage of key functions in electronic health records from 2005 to 2007: A statewide survey. *Journal of the American Medical Informatics Association* 16(4):465–470.

Star, S.L. and K. Ruhleder. 1996. Steps towards an ecology of infrastructure: Design and access for large information spaces. *Information Systems Research* (7):111–135.

Zhou, Li, C.S. Soran, C.A. Jenter, L.A. Volk, E.J. Orav, D.W. Bates, and S.R. Simon. 2009. The relationship between electronic health record use and quality of care over time. *Journal of the American Medical Informatics Association* 16(4):457–464.

Suggested Readings

Alsid, J. and J. Leviss. 2012 (March 3). Workforce Development Essential to Obama's Health Care IT Initiative. *Huffington Post*. http://www.huffingtonpost.com/julian-l-alssid-and-jonathan-a-leviss/workforce-development-ess_b_171556.html.

Daray, M. J. E. (2009). Negotiating electronic health record technology agreements. *The Health Lawyer* 22(2):53–160.

Fahrenholz, C.G., L.J. Smith, K. Tucker, and D. Warner. 2009. Plan B: A practical approach to downtime planning in medical practices. *Journal of AHIMA* 80(11):34–38.

Grabenbauer, L., R. Fraser, J. McClay, N. Woelfl, C. B. Thompson, J. Cambell, and J. Windle. 2011. Adoption of electronic health records. *Applied Clinical Informatics* 2(2):165–176.

Graham. J., D. Levick, and R. Schreiber R. 2010. AMDIS case conference: Intrusive medication safety alerts. *Applied Clinical Informatics* 1(1):68–78.

Grassley, C.E. 2010 (January 20). Grassley asks hospitals about experiences with federal health information technology program. Washington, DC: US Senate. http://grassley.senate.gov/news/Article.cfm?customel_dataPageID_1502=24867.

Institute for Healthcare Improvement. 2011. Failure Modes and Effects Analysis Tool. http://www.ihi.org/knowledge/Pages/Tools/FailureModesandEffectsAnalysisTool.aspx.

Institute of Medicine of the National Academies. 2012. Health IT and Patient Safety: Building safer systems for better care. Washington, DC: National Academies Press.

Jones, S.S., P.S. Heaton, R.S. Rudin, and E.C. Schneider. 2012. Unraveling the IT productivity paradox—lessons for health care. *New England Journal of Medicine* 366(24):2243–2245.

Keenan, G.M., E. Yakel, K. Dunn Lopez, D. Tschannen, and Y. Ford. 2012 (July 21). Challenges to nurses' efforts of retrieving, documenting and communicating patient care. *Journal of the American Medical Informatic Association*. doi:10.1136/amiajnl-2012-000894.

Keenan, G.M., E. Yakel, Y. Yao, D. Xu, L. Szalacha, J. Chen, A. Johnson, D. Tschannen, Y.B. Ford, and D.J. Wilkie. 2012 (July). Maintaining a consistent big picture: Meaningful use of a web-based POC EHR system. *International Journal of Nursing Knowledge* 23(3):119–33.

Kilbridge, P. 2003. Computer crash: Lessons from a system failure. *New England Journal of Medicine* 348(10):881–882.

Killelea, B.K., R. Kaushal, M. Cooper, G.J. Kuperman. 2007. To what extent do pediatricians accept computer-based dosing suggestions? *Pediatrics* 119(1):69–75.

Koppel, R. and D. Kreda. 2009. Health care information technology vendors "hold harmless" clause: implications for patients and clinicians. *Journal of the American Medical Association* 301(12):1276–1278.

Kuperman, G.J., A. Bobb, T.H. Payne, A.J. Avery, T.K. Gandhi, G. Burns, D.C. Classen, D.W. Bates. 2007. Medication-related clinical decision support in computerized provider order entry systems: A review. *Journal of the American Medical Informatics Association* 14(1):29–40.

Kuperman, G.J., R.M. Reichley, T.C. Bailey. 2006. Using commercial knowledge bases for clinical decision support; opportunities, hurdles, and recommendations. *Journal of the American Medical Informatics Association* 13(4):369–71.

Leviss, J. 2011. HIT or Miss: Studying failures to enable success. *Applied Clinical Informatics* 2(3):345–349.

Leviss, J., R. Kremsdorf, and M. Mohaideen. 2006. The CMIO—a new leader in healthcare. *Journal of the American Medical Informatics Association* 13(5):573–578.

Murff, H. and J. Kannry. 2001. Physician satisfaction with two order entry systems. *Journal of the American Medical Informatics Association* 8:499–509.

Obama, B. 2009 (February 24). President Obama's Address to Congress. The New York Times [Internet]. Available from http://www.nytimes.com/2009/02/24/us/politics/24obama-text.html.

Palmieri, P., L. Peterson, and L. Bedoya Corazzo. 2011. Technological iatrogenesis: The manifestation of inadequate organizational planning and the integration of health information technology. In J. A. Wolfe, H. Hanson, M. J. Moir, Friedman, L., & G. T. Savage, M. D. (Eds.), *Advances in Health Care Management* (Organizational Development in Healthcare, Vol. 10, pp. 287–312). Bingley, UK: Emerald Group Publishing.

Report by the Comptroller and Auditor General of the National Audit Office (United Kingdom): The National Programme for IT in the NHS: An update on the delivery of detailed care records systems. HC 888, Session 2010–2012, May 18, 2011.

Silow-Carroll, S., J. Edwards, and D. Rodin. 2012. Using electronic health records to improve quality and efficiency: The experiences of leading hospitals. Commonwealth Fund pub. 17:1–40.

Sittig, D. and H. Singh. 2012. Electronic health records and national patient-safety goals. *New England Journal of Medicine.* 367(19):1854–1860.

Terpenning, M., A. Berlin, and J. Graham. 2011. AMDIS case conference: Implementing electronic health records in a small subspecialty practice. *Applied Clinical Informatics* 2(2):158–164.

Additional Resources

General

The Standish Group. 1995. *Chaos Report*. http://net.educause.edu/ir/library/pdf/NCP08083B.pdf.

The Standish Group. 2001. Extreme CHAOS. http://www.cin.ufpe.br/~gmp/docs/papers/extreme_chaos2001.pdf.

Healthcare

Success and Failure Factors—Research Papers

Brender, J., E. Ammenwerth, P. Nykänen, and J. Talmon. 2006. Factors influencing success and failure of health informatics systems: A pilot Delphi study. *Methods of Information in Medicine* 45(1):125–136.

Heeks, R. 2006. Health information systems: Failure, success and improvisation. *International Journal of Medical Informatics* 75:125–137.

Kaplan, B. and K.D. Harris-Salamone. 2009. Health IT project success and failure: Recommendations from an AMIA workshop. *Journal American Medical Informatics Association* 16(3):291–299.

Ong, K. 2007. Why do projects fail? Chapter 16 in *Medical Informatics: An Executive Primer*. Edited by Ong, K. Chicago: HIMSS.

Paré, G., C. Sicotte, M. Jaana, and D. Girouard. 2008. Prioritizing the risk factors influencing the success of clinical information systems. *Methods of Information in Medicine* 47(3):251–259.

Van der Meijden, M.J., H.H. Tange, J. Troost, and A. Hasman. 2003. Determinants of success of inpatient clinical information systems: A literature review. *Journal of the American Medical Informatics Association* 10(3):235–243.

Success and Failure Factors—Practitioner Advice

Glaser, J. 2004 (October). Management's role in IT project failure. *Healthcare Financial Management*.

Glaser, J. 2005 (January). More on management's role in IT project failure. *Healthcare Financial Management*.

Examples

Research Case Studies and Analyses

Aarts, J. and M. Berg. 2006. Same system, different outcomes. *Methods of Information in Medicine* 45:53–61.

Aarts, J., H. Doorewaard, and M. Berg. 2004. Understanding implementation: The case of a computerized physician order entry systems in a large Dutch university medical center. *Journal of the American Medical Informatics Association* 11(3):207–216.

Beynon-Davies, P. 1995. Information systems 'failure': The case of the London ambulance service computer-aided despatch project. *European Journal of Information Systems* 4:171–184.

Beynon-Davies, P. and M. Lloyd-Williams. 1999. When health information systems fail. *Topics in Health Information Management* 19(4):66–79.

Brown, A.D. and M.R. Jones. 1998. Doomed to failure: Narratives of inevitability and conspiracy in a failed IS project. *Organization Studies* 19(1):73–88.

Dowling, A.F. 1980. Do hospital staff interfere with computer system implementation? *Health Care Management Review* 5:23–32.

House of Commons Public Accounts Committee. 2009 (January 27). *The National Programme for IT in the NHS: Progress since 2006.* London: The Stationery Office Ltd.

Lundsgaarde, H.P., P.J. Fischer, and D.J. Steele. 1981. *Human Problems in Computerized Medicine.* Lawrence, KS: The University of Kansas.

Massaro, T.A. 1993. Introducing physician order entry at a major academic medical center. 1: Impact on organizational culture and behavior. *Academic Medicine* 68(1):20–25.

Massaro, T.A. 1993. Introducing physician order entry at a major academic medical center. 2: Impact on medical education. *Academic Medicine* 68(1):25–30.

Sicotte, C., J.L. Denis, and P. Lehoux. 1998. The computer-based patient record: A strategic issue in process innovation. *Journal of Medical Systems* 22(6):431–443.

Sicotte, C., J.L. Denis, P. Lehoux, and F. Champagne. 1998. The computer-based patient record: Challenges towards timeless and spaceless medical practice. *Journal of Medical Systems* 22(4):237–256.

Southon, F.G.C., C. Sauer, and C.N.G. Dampney. 1997. Information technology in complex health services: Organizational impediments to successful technology transfer and diffusion. *Journal of the American Medical Informatics Association* 4:112–124.

van't Riet, A., M. Berg, F. Hiddema, and S. Kees. 2001. Meeting patients' needs with patient information systems: Potential benefits from qualitative research methods. *International Journal of Medical Informatics* 64:1–14.

Wells, S. and C. Bullen. 2008. A near miss: The importance of context in a public health informatics project in a New Zealand case study. *Journal of the American Medical Informatics Association* 15(5):701–704.

Useful Compilations

European Federation of Medical Informatics. 2009. Bad health informatics can kill. http://iig.umit.at/efmi/badinformatics.htm.

Silverstein, S. 2007. Sociotechnologic issues in clinical computing: Common examples of healthcare IT difficulties. http://www.ischool.drexel.edu/faculty/ssilverstein/cases/?loc=about.

Unintended Consequences

Ash, J., M. Berg, and E.W. Coiera. 2004. Some unintended consequences of information technology in health care: The nature of patient care information system-related errors. *Journal of the American Medical Informatics Association* 11(2):104–112.

Campbell, E, D. Sittig, J. Ash, K. Guappone, and R. Dykstra. 2006. Types of unintended consequences related to computerized provider order entry. *Journal of the American Medical Informatics Association* 13(5):547–56.

Harrison, M.I., R. Koppel, and S. Bar-Lev. 2007. Unintended consequences of information technologies in health care: An interactive sociotechnical analysis. *Journal of the American Medical Informatics Association* 14(5):542–549.

Errors

Han, Y.Y., J.A. Carcillo, S.T. Venkataraman, R.S. Clark, R.S. Watson, T.C. Mguyen, H. Bayir, and R.A. Orr. 2005. Unexpected increased mortality after implementation of a commercially sold computerized physician order entry system. *Pediatrics* 116(6):1506–1512.

Koppel, R., J.P. Metlay, A. Cohen, B. Abaluck, A.R. Localio, S.E. Kimmel, and B. L. Strom. 2005. Role of computerized physician order entry systems in facilitating medication errors. *Journal of the American Medical Association* 293(10):1197–1203.

Sustainability

Wetter, T. 2007. To decay is system: The challenges of keeping a health information system alive. *International Journal of Medical Informatics* 76S:S252–S260.

Workarounds

Koppel, R., T. Wetterneck, J.L. Telles, and B-T. Karsh. 2008. Workarounds to barcode medication administration systems: Their occurrences, causes, and threats to patient safety. *Journal of the American Medical Informatics Association* 15(4):408–423.

Vogelsmeier, A.A., J.R.B. Halbersleben, and J.R. Scott-Cawiezell. 2008. Technology implementation and workarounds in the nursing home. *Journal of the American Medical Informatics Association* 15(1):114–119.

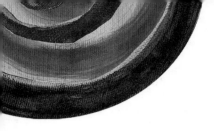

Index

Closed loop systems, 89
  for medications, 46
  "smart," 90
Closed-loop laboratory order management
    system, 75
CM. *See* Context management (CM)
CMIO. *See* Chief medical informatics officer
    (CMIO)
CMO. *See* Chief medical officer (CMO)
CMS. *See* Centers for Medicare and Medicaid
    Services (CMS)
CNIO. *See* Chief nursing informatics officer
    (CNIO)
Cognitive processes, 207
Collaboration
  in developing HIT application, 156, 201
  importance of, 63–67
Communication, 159, 161, 162, 165, 186
  among all users and stakeholders, 52,
    85, 133, 154
  among end-user community, health
    system management, and IT project
    team, 24
  among projects, 78
  bidirectional, 85
  channels of, 169, 170
  collaborative, conflicts between health
    system IT team and vendor team,
    95–96
  issues and emergencies, plan for, 168–70
  patterns, 207
  project team, 24
  protocols, 162
  risk mitigation and action plans of, 100
  between vendor and customer, 151
  verbal, 52
Community case studies
  adolescent confidentiality and pediatric
    PHR access, 191–95
  sharing information across a physician
    referral network, 185–90
  teaching module, 197–201
Community health center, custom EHR
    system designed for, 147–51
Community-based physicians, 189–90
Compatibility, 207
Complex medication lists, entry and
    reconciliation of, 26

Complex system implementations, 139
Comprehensive implementations, 139
Computer training courses, 40
Computer-based patient records, integration
    of, 129
Computerization movements, 207
Computerized physician order entry (CPOE),
    25–26, 107–11
  adoption of, 75
Computerized provider order entry (CPOE),
    16, 93, 113–17, 155, 178
  assessing progress of, 6
  go-live support for, 4, 5
  implementing, 3–7
  interfaces and medication errors in,
    43–46
  mandatory use of, 3–7
  order sets and, 121–27
  pilot of, 4–6
  political support for, 46
  usage growing for, 89
  user community incentives for, 6
  verbal communication reduced by, 52
Computer-savvy nurses, 38
Confidentiality concerns, PHR, 192, 195
Conflict avoidance behaviors, 24
Conflicting suboptimal practice
    patterns, 125
Congruence, 207
Consistent communication, 170
Context management (CM), 93
Contingency planning, importance of, 90
Contracts, vendor, 53
Cost overrun, 97–101
Cost weighing, 124
Cost-effective patient care, 126, 127
CPOE. *See* Computerized physician order
    entry (CPOE); Computerized provider
    order entry (CPOE)
Creatine Kinase (CPK), 122
Critical project resources, 39
Critical thinking, 206
CRM. *See* Customer relationship
    management (CRM)
Crystal Reports expert, 148
Cultures, merging healthcare system and
    university, 103–6
Custom development, 72, 77, 78